Understanding your
Eyes:
Cataracts,
Glaucoma and
Macular
Degeneration

Mr Robert Walters

Publis
in ass

© Family Doctor Publications 2003–9
Updated 2004, 2006, 2008, 2009

Acknowledgements: The author would like to acknowledge the
expert help and advice given by his colleagues Christopher Blyth
and James Morgan, and to thank his wife, Jane, for her support
and encouragement. Thanks also to his secretary, Kathryn Murphy,
for her help in organisation and word processing.

Family Doctor Publications, PO Box 4664, Poole, Dorset BH15 1NN

ISBN-13: 978-1-903474-40-2
ISBN-10: 1-903474-40-X

Contents

Introduction 1

Your eyes and how they work 10

Common sight problems 23

Cataracts 34

Cataract surgery 44

Glaucoma 70

Surgery for open-angle glaucoma 88

Macular degeneration 98

Registration as blind or partially sighted 117

Useful addresses 123

Index 136

Your pages 147

About the author

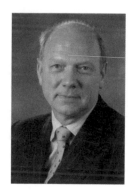

Mr Robert Walters is a Consultant Eye Surgeon at the University Hospital of Wales, having trained in London and Southampton. He is an Examiner and previous Regional Adviser for the Royal College of Ophthalmologists. He is also a previous NHS Clinical Director and is currently Lead Clinician. He is on the Board of Directors of ORBIS International, a charity dedicated to the prevention and treatment of blindness in developing countries. He has been the Chairman of the Board of Trustees of ORBIS UK since 2008. His practice involves general ophthalmology, cataract surgery and the treatment of disorders of eye movement.

Introduction

Some deterioration is normal

As you get older, it's natural for your eyesight to deteriorate slightly and for you to need reading glasses or stronger distance glasses, depending on your eyesight. However, there are also some specific eye conditions that can affect older people and it is important for you to be aware of these.

Conditions of which you should be aware

Cataracts, glaucoma and macular degeneration are the most common causes of poor sight in the UK. Each one predominantly affects people of middle age and beyond, and if detected early there is a better chance of preventing serious loss of sight.

Many people with visual difficulties in later life are unnecessarily frightened that they are going to experience progressive visual loss that will curtail their lifestyle or threaten their independence.

This book will provide you with comprehensive and simple explanations of common eye conditions and of their causes and treatments. It is intended to supplement information and advice given to you by your doctor, optometrist (optician) and hospital eye specialist (ophthalmologist). If you think that you have an eye problem, you should seek professional help.

Cataracts

This condition is a clouding of the lens of the eye (see page 34) and results in deterioration of vision. Cataracts are estimated to affect over a million people in the UK alone. They can be treated surgically; cataract surgery is in fact by far the most common operation performed in British eye units, with more than 300,000 operations every year.

Cataract surgery has been carried out for thousands of years and it is known that the ancient Egyptians commonly performed operations using a technique called couching. This involved introducing a sharp implement, such as a thorn, into the eye in order to dislocate a mature cataractous lens away from the visual axis or to pierce it so that it is mostly reabsorbed. This procedure remained the principal form of treatment for cataracts until the late nineteenth century.

Lens replacement

Over the last 50 years, astonishing advances have been made, the most notable of which has been the introduction of a surgical procedure called intraocular lens implantation, which permanently replaces the cataractous lens with a lens implant. Patients no longer need to wear the thick glasses previously necessary after surgery. Indeed, after their operation, many do not need any glasses for everyday distance vision.

The pioneering work with intraocular lens implantation was carried out by a British eye surgeon,

Mr Harold Ridley, in London in 1949 using shaped Perspex. This remarkable advance followed the observation of the RAF pilots during World War II who suffered perforating eye injuries from the shattered Perspex canopies of their planes. Mr Ridley noted that the Perspex inside the eye did not cause any inflammation because it was inert.

He reasoned that, if Perspex could be made into a lens shape, it could be implanted in the eye to restore the sight of those whose natural lens had been removed because of a cataract. Perspex intraocular lens implants are still used today, although other materials, such as acrylic, are also used. Harold Ridley was knighted, in recognition of his contribution, in 1999 shortly before he died.

Recent advances in surgical technique

Until the late 1970s, everyone undergoing cataract surgery had to stay in hospital for five days or longer. The surgery carried such great risks that it was considered only if the cataract was causing severe visual loss.

These days, technical innovations such as microscopic surgery, advanced materials and instrument design, and surgery using small incisions mean that most cataract operations are carried out as day-case procedures and the chances of success are very high. People no longer have to wait until their vision is severely impaired to have a cataract operation but can proceed to surgery when their symptoms are beginning to affect aspects of their everyday life, such as driving or reading.

Glaucoma

The term 'glaucoma' (see page 70) covers a variety of

conditions characterised by high pressure within the eye and a gradual loss of the peripheral (side) field of vision. It is estimated that there are 300,000 people in the UK with varying degrees of glaucoma, although most forms do not occur until after the age of 40 years and there are no symptoms until the late stages.

Most optometrists in the UK carry out a comprehensive screening programme for glaucoma as part of the routine eye examination. If you are over the age of 40, your optometrist will measure your eye pressure using a simple procedure.

If the pressure is higher than normal, he or she can refer you to your doctor to be considered for a consultation with a hospital eye specialist (ophthalmologist). The condition can be treated and, if diagnosed early on, there is a good chance of preventing serious visual loss.

Macular degeneration

This is a condition that usually affects only people older than 60 years, and thus is known as 'age-related' macular degeneration (see page 100). There are other forms of the disease that affect younger people, but these are rare and beyond the scope of this book. Macular degeneration can cause difficulties with your central (reading) vision because of changes in the most sensitive part of your retina called the macula.

Age-related macular degeneration is surprisingly common; it is estimated that 10 per cent of people aged between 65 and 75 are affected to some degree, rising to 30 per cent of those older than 75.

Wearing stronger glasses and using other visual aids can help many of those with the disease. Even in the worst form of the disease, where the central vision is severely impaired, the peripheral (side) vision is not usually affected so you can still see your way around. People who have age-related macular degeneration gain great comfort from the knowledge that they will never go blind or lose their sight completely from this condition. There has been a recent advance in the treatment of one type of macular degeneration (the wet variety) and this is described later.

Links between the eye conditions

Although cataracts, glaucoma and macular degeneration are not interrelated they can coexist because they are all conditions that affect people as they get older. If you have macular degeneration and cataracts, then removal of the cataracts can still lead to an improvement in vision, although the degree of improvement depends on the severity of the macular degenerative changes and the cataracts.

Usually the cataractous lens has to interfere significantly with vision before removal would be recommended for patients with severe macular degeneration. Your optometrist may also be able to help with advice on this issue, but a consultation with and examination by the hospital eye specialist (ophthalmologist) will provide definitive advice.

Glaucoma and macular degeneration, although not strictly interrelated, are both more common in people who are short-sighted (myopes) and therefore it is particularly important that these people visit their optometrists every one to two years for a check-up.

What are the responsibilities of the different eye professionals?
Ophthalmologist (ophthalmic surgeon)
An ophthalmologist is a qualified doctor of medicine

who has undergone considerable further postgraduate hospital training in the diagnosis and treatment (both medical and surgical) of eye disease.

This training to consultant level takes approximately 10 years after obtaining the basic medical degree. All hospital consultants have obtained specialist postgraduate qualifications including a Fellowship of the Royal College of Ophthalmologists in the UK or its equivalent from Scotland or overseas. To practise as consultants suitably qualified doctors have to be on the 'specialist register' with the General Medical Council.

Many of the older ophthalmologists will also have qualified as fellows of the Royal College of Surgeons of England, Edinburgh or Glasgow as this was the usual qualification obtained before the formation of the College of Ophthalmologists (later given the 'Royal' prefix) in 1986.

Optometrist

This term was introduced in the 1980s to distinguish between more highly qualified opticians and dispensing opticians (see below). An optometrist has obtained a professional degree in optometry and is trained in refraction, dispensing of glasses and the diagnosis of basic eye diseases.

They do not carry out surgery or prescribe medications other than simple eye lubricants. An optometrist will carry out eye examinations at the high-street optician. They are represented by the College of Optometrists and the regulatory and disciplinary body of optometrists (and dispensing opticians) is the General Optical Council of the UK. There are about 11,000 optometrists in the UK.

Dispensing optician

A dispensing optician is qualified to dispense glasses but not to carry out the refraction tests necessary to determine the power of the lenses within them. Dispensing opticians are not as highly qualified as optometrists but make a significant contribution to optometric practice. There are about 8,600 dispensing opticians in the UK.

Nurse practitioners

Increasing numbers of specially qualified higher-grade nurses are employed in hospital eye departments in the UK. These are termed 'nurse practitioners' and usually have a specialist nursing qualification in ophthalmology (Diploma in Ophthalmic Nursing).

These nurses make up an important part of the ophthalmic service and have many roles. For example, ophthalmic casualty nurses treat simple eye conditions such as corneal abrasions, glaucoma nurses measure intraocular pressures and carry out field tests, and treatment nurses are involved in minor operations such as removing lid cysts.

Orthoptists

This is one of the professions allied to medicine (PAMs) and orthoptists are qualified in the study and treatment of eye movement conditions such as squints. Although these make up the bulk of their work, in many departments they also carry out glaucoma screening, visual field testing and sometimes ophthalmic photography. There are approximately 1,000 qualified orthoptists in the UK.

Hospital eye department doctors

Within the hospital the leading ophthalmologists are the consultants. However, you will not always be seen by him or her; you may be seen by one of the other staff. These are divided into the training-grade staff, who are training to become consultant ophthalmologists, and non-consultant ophthalmic medical staff.

All non-consultant and training-grade doctors are under the supervision of the consultants who carry the ultimate clinical responsibility for patients under their care.

The hospital eye service is usually provided by a combination of consultants, doctors undergoing postgraduate training and non-consultant grades, often in association with nurse practitioners, orthoptists and occasionally optometrists.

KEY POINTS

■ Cataracts are common in elderly people but vision can easily be restored with cataract surgery, which nowadays is a straightforward and safe procedure

■ Glaucoma is a silent condition that causes a gradual loss of peripheral vision. Your optometrist/optician will screen you for glaucoma when you have an eye test so that sight-saving treatment can be commenced early

■ Macular degeneration causes central or visual loss but never causes blindness

Your eyes and how they work

Eyes are very complex organs

Vision is truly the king of all the senses. Your eyes are among the most highly specialised and sensitive organs of your body. The eye, optic nerve and brain work together to produce an image. To enable you to see, light rays must pass through the cornea (the front of the eye), pupil (the black hole) and lens to be focused on your retina (at the back of your eye – see page 19). An electrical signal is generated in the retina and passed along the optic nerve to specialist parts of the brain where the image is interpreted.

Protection for your eyes

The eyes are roughly spherical and they sit in the bony eye sockets of the orbits. The eyeballs are cushioned with a layer of fat and held in place by a series of muscles, which also allow movement (see page 13). Only a small part of the eye is visible; the rest of the sphere is within the skull. The visible part of your eyes is further protected by your eyelids, which provide thick protective coats and lashes that help to prevent foreign bodies such as dirt and dust entering your eye.

Eyes are lubricated with tears

The eyelids keep the eyes lubricated by spreading a special liquid (tears) over the surface of your eyes at regular intervals. The film of tears is produced in the lacrimal glands, which lie just above your eyeballs in the outer upper part of your eye sockets. Tears prevent your eyes from drying out and protect them from infections.

Tears help protect the eyes

Tears are produced by the lacrimal glands. They prevent the eyes from drying out and protect them from infection, and drain away through the nose.

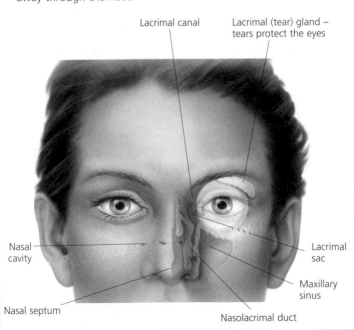

Lacrimal canal

Lacrimal (tear) gland – tears protect the eyes

Nasal cavity

Lacrimal sac

Maxillary sinus

Nasal septum

Nasolacrimal duct

The tears are spread by the blinking action of your eyelids and drain away into two canals (tear ducts) at the inner part of your eyelids and then through a fine tube to your nose.

We notice tears only when excess liquid is produced, for example, when we cry. The tears drain away through your nose which is one reason why crying can block your nose. If the tears are reduced in volume or the quality of the tear film is poor, your eyes will feel dry and uncomfortable. You can buy artificial tears at the chemist, which can soothe dry eyes but never completely replace the natural tear film.

Eye movements

Your eyes swivel in their sockets using six delicate muscles attached to the outside of each eye. These muscles control the position of the eyes so accurately that, when you are reading a book, they can pinpoint successive lines of text in less than one-hundredth of a second.

The movement of the eye muscles is controlled by three nerves that come directly from the brain (the third, fourth and sixth cranial nerves). The front surface of the eye has a clear central portion (the cornea) and the rest is covered by a waterproof protective layer (the conjunctiva) that extends from the edges of the cornea and covers around one-third of the eyeball.

Beneath the conjunctiva lies the sclera, a tough fibrous layer that provides the main structural wall of your eyeball. The sclera and conjunctiva form the 'white of the eye'.

Inside the eyes

The eye is very complex. The cornea is the clear central portion across the front of the eye. It is strong and

How eyes move

Each eye swivels in its eye socket using six delicate and very precise muscles attached to the outside of the eyeball.

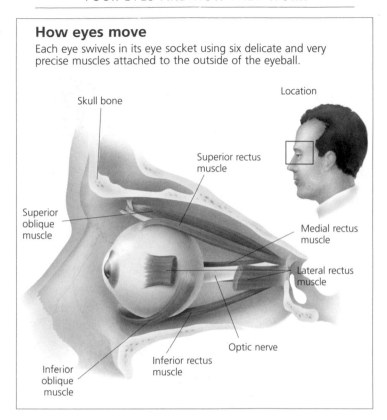

Location

Skull bone

Superior rectus muscle

Superior oblique muscle

Medial rectus muscle

Lateral rectus muscle

Optic nerve

Inferior rectus muscle

Inferior oblique muscle

allows light to pass through it. The cornea carries out most of the focusing of the eye. It refracts (bends) light entering your eye on to the lens behind the pupil, which then fine tunes the focusing of the image so that it falls accurately on the retina. The iris – the coloured tissue around the pupil – is made up of fine layers of muscle with the pupil as a central hole.

Pupils adapt to light levels

Pupils are highly sensitive to light, dilating in darkness,

The structure of the eye

Each eye is roughly spherical, but only a small part is visible. The eyes are protected by the eye sockets in the skull and surrounded by a layer of fat.

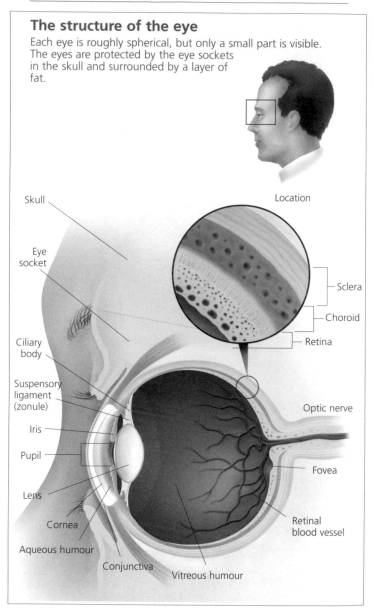

Location

Skull

Eye socket

Ciliary body

Suspensory ligament (zonule)

Iris

Pupil

Lens

Cornea

Aqueous humour

Conjunctiva

Vitreous humour

Sclera

Choroid

Retina

Optic nerve

Fovea

Retinal blood vessel

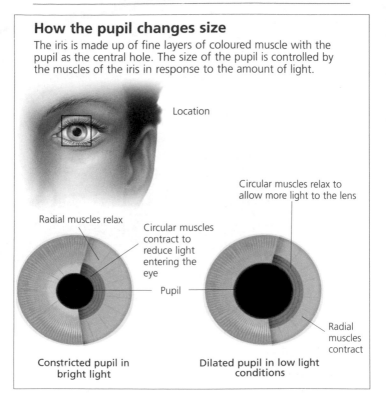

How the pupil changes size

The iris is made up of fine layers of coloured muscle with the pupil as the central hole. The size of the pupil is controlled by the muscles of the iris in response to the amount of light.

Location

Radial muscles relax

Circular muscles contract to reduce light entering the eye

Circular muscles relax to allow more light to the lens

Pupil

Radial muscles contract

Constricted pupil in bright light

Dilated pupil in low light conditions

or when you are excited, to allow more light into the eyes, but quickly constrict to protect them in bright light. The size of the pupil is controlled by the muscles of the iris. The colour of the iris, which determines the colour of your eyes, is inherited from your parents or grandparents.

Belladonna eye drops (derived from the deadly nightshade plant and now called atropine) were used by ladies in the court of Louis XIV of France to dilate (widen) their pupils because they believed that it made them look more beautiful. Hence the name 'bella donna' which means 'beautiful lady'.

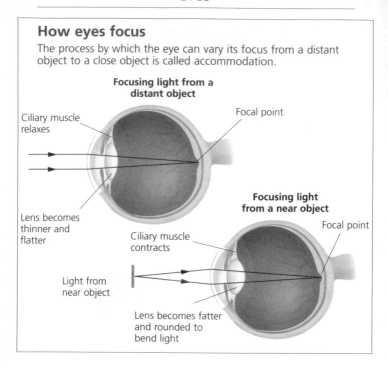

How eyes focus

The process by which the eye can vary its focus from a distant object to a close object is called accommodation.

Focusing light from a distant object

Ciliary muscle relaxes

Focal point

Lens becomes thinner and flatter

Focusing light from a near object

Ciliary muscle contracts

Focal point

Light from near object

Lens becomes fatter and rounded to bend light

Front chamber of the eye

The eye is made up of two fluid-filled chambers. The front chamber, between the lens and the cornea, is filled with a liquid called aqueous humour that bathes and nourishes this part of the eye. The fluid circulates continually. It is produced behind the iris by the ciliary body. The fluid passes around the inside of the eye and through the pupil to leave the eye mainly through a 'drainage angle' in the trabecular meshwork, which lies between the base of the iris and the cornea.

The lens

This lies behind the pupil and is suspended by a series of very fine threads (the zonules). These threads can tighten or loosen, under the control of a muscle (ciliary muscle) to which they are attached, enabling the lens to become fatter or slimmer. The muscle is circular and shaped like a tyre's inner tube and the zonules are attached to the inside surface.

When the muscle contracts the size of the circle becomes smaller and the zonules relax. The zonules are also attached to the lens so that, when the zonules relax, the lens can also relax and become fatter in shape, increasing its focusing power. This process is called 'accommodation' and enables the eye to vary its focus from a distant object to one that is closer.

Thus, for looking at near objects (such as reading a book) the 'ciliary muscle' as it is called contracts and allows the lens to become fatter, bending the light rays more to focus the image on the retina. Conversely, for viewing objects in the distance the ciliary muscle relaxes, thereby tightening the zonules and stretching the lens, which will then bend the light rays less and focus the light once again on the retina.

The lens is shaped like a Smartie sweet and has an outer 'capsule' and an inner 'nucleus' and 'cortex'. It is translucent and has no direct blood supply because it gets the nutrients and oxygen that it requires from the fluid in which it is bathed (the aqueous humour).

The inner chamber

The second fluid-filled chamber lies behind the lens. It is large and filled with a clear jelly-like substance called the 'vitreous humour'. This is important in the formation of your eye in the uterus (particularly the lens) but has no known significant function after birth.

In middle age and beyond the vitreous humour tends to shrink and lose some of its clarity, forming

Anatomy of vision

The function of the components of the eye in vision, from light entering the pupil to the nerve impulse to the brain.

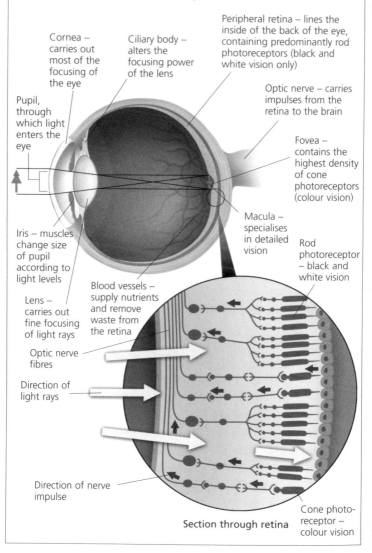

Cornea – carries out most of the focusing of the eye

Ciliary body – alters the focusing power of the lens

Peripheral retina – lines the inside of the back of the eye, containing predominantly rod photoreceptors (black and white vision only)

Optic nerve – carries impulses from the retina to the brain

Pupil, through which light enters the eye

Fovea – contains the highest density of cone photoreceptors (colour vision)

Iris – muscles change size of pupil according to light levels

Macula – specialises in detailed vision

Rod photoreceptor – black and white vision

Lens – carries out fine focusing of light rays

Blood vessels – supply nutrients and remove waste from the retina

Optic nerve fibres

Direction of light rays

Direction of nerve impulse

Cone photo-receptor – colour vision

Section through retina

'floaters' that you can see, particularly in bright light looking at a plain light-coloured surface. The vitreous humour does not circulate like the aqueous humour.

Light-sensitive retina

The retina lines the inside of the back of the eye. It is a wafer-thin layer containing about 130 million light-sensitive cells called photoreceptors (in the form of rods and cones).

The rod photoreceptors (about 123 million) lie in the peripheral (outer) part of the retina and deal with black and white vision. They are sensitive to low-intensity light, but cannot differentiate between colours, which is why objects appear to lose colour at night.

Colour vision is served by the cone photoreceptors, which are fewer in number (about seven million) and work best in high-intensity light. There are three types; each type responds to a different primary colour (red, blue or green). Cones are concentrated in the centre of the retina (the macula). The macula specialises in detailed vision – reading and recognising faces.

Cone defects

Some people are born with mild defects in one or more of the three kinds of cones and this leads to colour blindness. For example, eight per cent of men are red/green colour blind, being unable to distinguish clearly between red and green. This can mean that they cannot clearly tell the difference between a red and green traffic light, but can drive safely because they know that the top light means stop and the bottom light means go.

The optic nerve

Nerve fibres connect the photoreceptors to the brain. The millions of nerve connections from the retina collect together in the optic nerve; there are two optic nerves, one for each eye. At the base of the brain, the two optic nerves join and then divide into separate channels (tracts). After further processing, the nerves pass to the occipital cortex, a specialist part of the brain that interprets the visual signals as images.

How you see

The visual system can be likened to two video cameras (the eyes) connected to a computer (the brain) by connecting electrical cables (the optic nerves). The cornea and lens form the focusing mechanism of the camera. They focus light to form an image that is projected on to the retina at the back of the eye.

The photoreceptors in the retina translate the light energy into an electrical signal, which is transmitted along the optic nerves to a specialist part of the brain (the visual cortices). The picture on the retina is upside down and back to front. However, the brain is programmed to interpret this image the right way up. The visual cortices interpret electrical signals received from the eyes and translate them into the image that we see. This immensely complicated process is only partially understood.

Sight is such an important sense that a large proportion of the brain is dedicated to interpreting what we see. Interestingly, the left side of the brain deals with images from the right visual field (in both eyes) and the right side of the brain with images from the left visual field. Therefore, people who have a stroke affecting the visual cortex on one side of their

Field of vision

The left side of the brain processes images from the right visual field (in both eyes) and vice versa.

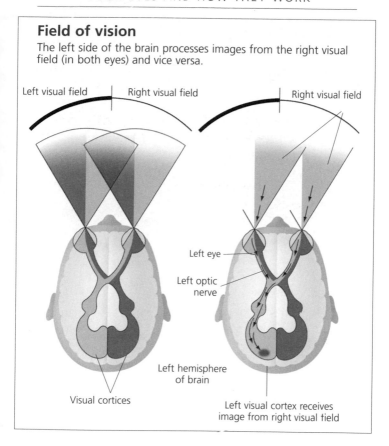

Left visual field | Right visual field

Right visual field

Left eye

Left optic nerve

Left hemisphere of brain

Visual cortices

Left visual cortex receives image from right visual field

brain find that the opposite half of their visual field is blanked out in both eyes.

KEY POINTS

- Your eyes are highly specialised, complicated organs

- Each eye works like a camera: light rays pass through your pupil and are focused by your lens and cornea on to your retina

- Your retina contains millions of light-sensitive cells

Common sight problems

Normal sight variations

Many people have otherwise healthy eyes, apart from refractive errors that develop in childhood. For example, in some people, the image does not naturally focus on the retina, and these people are said to be either long-sighted (hypermetropic) or short-sighted (myopic). Others may see a distorted image as a result of astigmatism.

These are common problems that can be readily diagnosed during routine eye tests and can usually be corrected by wearing glasses or contact lenses. In addition, ageing can also affect your eyes, making it progressively more difficult for you to see close up (a sight problem called 'presbyopia'). Again this can be treated with glasses.

Importance of eye tests

Regular eye examinations should be part of your normal health regime from childhood so that your eyes can be examined internally and externally. In this way any refractive errors can be treated and early signs of health problems detected.

What happens in an eye examination?

This is a simple and painless procedure normally carried out by an optometrist. It involves testing your visual acuity, an examination of the eye with a microscope and a measurement of the pressure within your eye (intraocular pressure).

An eye examination typically takes 20 to 30 minutes and is usually combined with a refraction test (testing for glasses). Your eye movement and coordination will also be assessed. If your vision is becoming blurred because of refractive errors these can be simply corrected with a pair of glasses. If the examination by the optometrist gives rise to a suspicion of eye disease (such as cataracts or glaucoma), then he or she can refer you to a hospital eye specialist (ophthalmologist). This referral is usually coordinated with your doctor.

Visual acuity tests

Your vision is measured using a standardised back-lit chart (a Snellen chart). This test is carried out at a standard distance of six metres (albeit sometimes using a mirror). If you have normal vision you should be able to read the standard six-metre line at six metres away and your visual acuity would then be described as 6/6.

If your vision is reduced, you may be able to read only the larger letters above the six-metre line, for example, those that a person with 'normal vision' would be able to read at a distance of nine metres away. Your visual acuity would then be described as 6/9. Similarly, if you were able to read only the top

Snellen eye test chart

This is an example of the type of chart used by your optometrist; it is for illustration only and is of no use for eye testing.

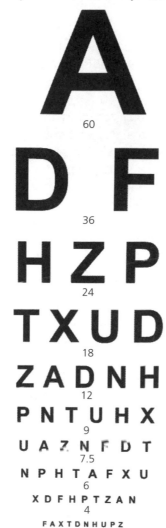

A
60

D F
36

H Z P
24

T X U D
18

Z A D N H
12

P N T U H X
9

U A Z N F D T
7.5

N P H T A F X U
6

X D F H P T Z A N
4

F A X T D N H U P Z

letter on the chart six metres away (which someone with 'normal' vision would be able to read 60 metres away), your visual acuity would be described as 6/60 and would be poor.

The metric system is used in the vast majority of countries throughout the world but in North America they have persisted in the use of feet rather than metres and so normal visual acuity of 6/6 in the UK would be described as 20/20 in North America.

Snellen chart vision testing is an extremely helpful standard method that is used throughout the world. However, it does not take into account other aspects of visual function, for example, contrast sensitivity and glare. If necessary more complex measurements can be carried out in specialist eye departments.

Health checks

As well as eye diseases, signs of other health problems such as high blood pressure and diabetes can be picked up at a routine eye test because it can show changes in the retina. If detected early enough, these conditions can be treated and managed effectively before complications such as sight loss can develop. It is therefore a sensible precaution to have an eye examination at least every two years. All eye examinations by the optician/optometrist for people aged 60 and over and 18 or under are free of charge. Free eye tests are also available on the NHS to other groups of people, including those with diabetes and glaucoma, people aged 40 and over who are the parent/brother/sister/child of someone with glaucoma, and those who are blind or partially sighted.

Refraction test

This is when the optometrist tests you for glasses.
It usually involves two stages:

1 **Objective test:** the first is an objective test using a
   'retinoscope' to shine a slit-shaped beam of light
   into your eye and the optometrist puts corrective
   lenses in front of your eye until any refractive error is
   neutralised.
2 **Subjective test:** this is followed by a subjective test
   in which lenses are put into a frame in front of your
   eyes and small changes are made to the lenses
   while you are asked whether your vision is better or
   worse with these changes.

The initial refraction test is carried out for distance
vision and then different lenses are used to test close-
up vision until both distance vision and near vision are
clear with the appropriate lenses.

Types of lens

If you need glasses for distance vision only then distance
glasses alone will be supplied. Likewise if you need only
reading glasses, these will be prescribed. However, if
you need glasses for both near and distance vision,
then separate reading and distance glasses, or bifocal
lenses (containing both types of lens), can be supplied.

Varifocal lenses are also available. These are graded
lenses that allow people to see in the distance through
the top part of the lens. The lens then becomes
progressively more powerful in the lower portions to
facilitate clear vision at middle distances and close-up
vision. Varifocal lenses have become more sophisticated
recently and are increasingly popular.

Trifocal lenses are available that consist of a three-part lens within the glasses, one for distance, one for middle distance and one for near. However, they have largely been replaced by Varifocal lenses.

Eye care in the UK

An optometrist will be able to check your vision, prescribe glasses if necessary and carry out a routine screening of your eyes. A recent change in the law has allowed optometrists to prescribe some broad-spectrum antibiotic eyedrops and ointment (chloramphenicol), and many drops and ointments are now used for initial diagnosis and sometimes treatment of basic eye conditions such as dry eyes. Optometrists also screen patients during a routine eye test for conditions such as glaucoma.

Your doctor can also give you a simple examination of your eyes, visual system and eye movements if disease is suspected.

Many general practice groups have specialist doctors with added training in monitoring conditions such as diabetes, who will be able to examine your retina for signs of this disease. If eye disease is suspected or has been found, you will be referred to a consultant ophthalmologist within the hospital eye service.

Specialist medical eye training in Britain is sophisticated and carried out to the highest standard. You can be confident that the hospital eye department will be well equipped and staffed by well-trained doctors, nurses and other staff. Many of the bigger hospital eye departments in the UK have supra-specialist eye consultants who, in addition to a general knowledge of eye conditions and treatments, have a specialist interest in branches of ophthalmology such as eye movement disorders (squints), glaucoma, retinal disease, oculoplastic disorders and many others.

Treating refractive errors

Refractive errors are often inherited or develop in childhood, although some develop with age.

Long-sightedness (hypermetropia)

If you are long-sighted, seeing close up may take more effort and can trigger headaches and blurred vision. In long-sightedness the image of a nearby object is formed behind your retina, rather than on it. This is either because your eyeball is too short or occasionally because your cornea is not curved enough. Most people are born mildly long-sighted but do not need glasses because they can focus through their long-sightedness, which also gradually reduces in the first 10 years of life.

People who are very long-sighted require glasses from childhood, although the strength of these may reduce during their teenage years before levelling off. People who are long-sighted in childhood need reading glasses at an earlier age. Long-sightedness can be corrected with a lens that refracts (bends) the light more (a positive-powered convex lens) so that it focuses accurately on your retina.

Short-sightedness (myopia)

If you are short-sighted, the opposite applies. You can see nearby objects easily, but looking at distant objects (for example, road signs) is more difficult. In short-sightedness the light from a distant object is focused in front of your retina. This is because either your eyeball is too long or, less frequently, your cornea is too curved. Short-sightedness usually develops in childhood

Lens correction for refractive errors

By placing a concave (curved inwards) or convex (curved outwards) lens in front of the eyes, the path of light from an object can be redirected so that it focuses on the retina, thus correcting vision.

1. Lenses for long-sightedness (hypermetropia)

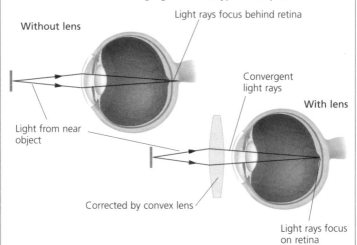

Light rays focus behind retina

Without lens

Convergent light rays

With lens

Light from near object

Corrected by convex lens

Light rays focus on retina

2. Lenses for short-sightedness (myopia)

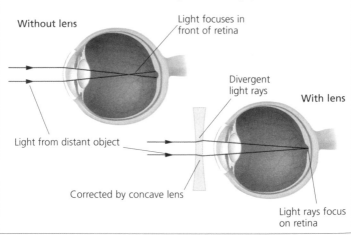

Light focuses in front of retina

Without lens

Divergent light rays

With lens

Light from distant object

Corrected by concave lens

Light rays focus on retina

(before the age of 20) and tends to stabilise in adulthood. It can be corrected by wearing glasses or contact lenses, with a negative-powered concave lens to focus the image on your retina.

People who are short-sighted often do not require reading glasses in later years (unlike the rest of the population) because they find that they can read by taking their glasses off. Some people prefer to have bifocal or Varifocal lenses so that they do not have to change their glasses for reading.

Astigmatism

If you have astigmatism, your cornea may be curved more in one direction than the other (shaped more like a rugby ball than a football) or your lens may bend the light unequally. You may notice that objects are blurred or out of focus. Astigmatism is usually inherited and may be present at birth, although it can also develop from a corneal scar or from surgery (for example, for cataracts). Glasses or contact lenses can be made to correct this abnormality.

Laser surgery for refractive errors

Detailed discussion about this topic is beyond the scope of this book but there has been increasing interest in laser surgery for the correction of a variety of refractive errors. Relatively low degrees of short-sightedness (up to six dioptres) can be corrected with laser treatment and recent advances have led to successful correction of low degrees of long-sightedness and astigmatism. However, you should bear in mind that all these refractive errors can be corrected with glasses or contact lenses and that laser treatment is a form of surgery, which, as such, carries a small risk of permanent damage to the eyes.

If you are contemplating laser treatment for refractive error, seek advice from an ophthalmologist or optometrist first. You can get information from the Royal College of Ophthalmologists (see page 130).

When cataract surgery is performed both short-sightedness and long-sightedness can be corrected by the use of a tailor-made lens implant in the eye. This should be discussed with the consultant ophthalmologist before cataract surgery.

Ageing and your eyes

As you get older, the lenses in your eyes may lose flexibility and you may find that it gradually becomes more difficult to focus on close objects. Many people notice their near sight deteriorating from around 40 years of age. This is presbyopia and is a natural part of ageing. It is not a disease and cannot be prevented, but it is easily corrected with reading glasses.

KEY POINTS

- It is important to have regular eye examinations to assess your sight and check for other health problems such as high blood pressure or diabetes

- If you are long-sighted, you cannot see close-up objects very clearly; if you are short-sighted, the opposite applies

- In astigmatism, your cornea is warped and objects seem blurred

- As you get older, your lenses lose flexibility, causing presbyopia

Cataracts

Cataracts are common

If you have been told by your doctor or optometrist that you have a cataract, you are not alone. Cataracts affect over half of all people aged over 65; they are often slow growing and may take many months or years to affect your vision significantly. Almost all cases of cataract can be treated successfully and modern cataract surgery is a relatively simple process, often requiring only one day in hospital.

What is a cataract?

Normally, the lens in the eye, which lies behind the pupil, is clear or transparent. It helps to focus light rays on to the retina at the back of the eye. If you have a cataract, however, your lens is cloudy (opaque) to varying degrees. This stops enough light from reaching your retina and the resulting picture is dull and fuzzy.

What causes a cataract?

Cataracts have many different causes. They can be congenital, age related, or the result of an eye injury or condition such as diabetes, or the long-term use of some drugs, for example, corticosteroids; also there can be other factors. There are also several different type of cataract (see pages 36–8).

Developmental problems

A few people are born with cataracts, known as congenital cataracts. They may be caused by disease during pregnancy, such as an infection, for example German measles (rubella). Fortunately, such cataracts are rare in the UK, although when they do occur they can sometimes substantially interfere with a baby's vision.

If a baby is born with significant cataracts, he or she can be successfully operated upon in a similar way to adults with cataracts but the resulting vision is not always good. All babies in the UK are screened for congenital cataracts as part of their health and development checks. These may show up as a white pupil or poor 'red reflex' in the pupil.

Many congenital cataracts are mild and inherited (rather than being related to a disease or infection), and consist of blue or white dots scattered throughout the lens. This type of congenital cataract seldom interferes with the normal development of vision in childhood and usually remains unchanged throughout life.

Age-related cataracts

By far the most common cause of cataracts in the western world is the ageing process and, if we live long enough, most of us will develop cataracts to some extent. As you get older, normal changes occur in the proteins in the lens, causing it to harden and lose its elasticity. These proteins may also clump together and form a cataract.

Cataracts caused by trauma

Severe injury, or trauma, such as a blow to the eye or a more severe eye injury, intense heat or chemical burns, can damage the lens of your eye, leading to the development of a cataract. This can occur at any age.

Diseases and other causes of cataracts

Some diseases such as diabetes mellitus (both the insulin-dependent and tablet/diet-controlled varieties, that is types 1 and 2) can cause significant lens opacities. However, these usually occur later in life and after the diabetes has been present for many years.

Some drugs (particularly corticosteroids), if used for a considerable period of time, can also cause cataracts. There is no set pattern for the development of these cataracts but, in general, the higher the dose the greater the likelihood of cataract development.

Other factors that have been implicated in the development of cataracts include long-standing inflammation in the eye (uveitis or iritis) and ionising radiation such as radiation from nuclear fission or X-rays. Cataracts are also associated with poor levels of nutrition particularly in developing countries, but this is not a significant factor in the western world.

Long-term exposure to high levels of sunshine (particularly ultraviolet light) and smoking have also been cited as causes. However, these last two factors remain controversial.

Types of cataract

There are many different forms of cataract, but there are three types that commonly occur as part of the ageing process. Sometimes people may have more than one form.

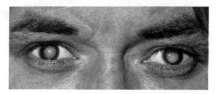

This shows the typical cloudy appearance of eyes affected by mature cataracts.

Nuclear sclerotic cataract

This cataract causes clouding of the central nucleus of the lens. Initially yellow, it becomes browner as the cataract matures. It can cut out the light and cause blurred vision, and colours appear much duller. This cataract develops gradually; affected people may not notice loss of vision until late on. The loss of colour vision results in the false assumption that home furnishings are dull or dirty, and people replace them with strident colours to compensate.

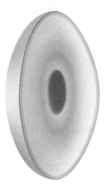

Typical appearance of affected lens in cross-section.

Cortical cataract

This type of cataract is characterised by whitish spoke-like patches on the outer part of the lens. It may not affect vision for many years, although you may be sensitive to or dazzled by very bright light. A common symptom is image ghosting, or double vision.

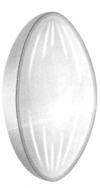

Typical appearance of affected lens in cross-section.

Posterior subcapsular cataract

This mainly affects the outer layer at the back of the lens and causes yellow or white clouding of the lens. This cataract can lead to early deterioration of vision; sometimes sight is significantly reduced within a few months. It can be linked with ageing but also to other conditions such as diabetes, or to long-term steroid use.

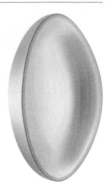

Typical appearance of affected lens in cross-section.

Symptoms of cataracts

Cataracts are usually found in both eyes, but they are often not at the same stage of development (asymmetrically advanced), so that the vision in one of your eyes may be worse than that of the other. The severity of cataracts varies greatly. Some people may not be aware that a cataract is developing because it can develop at the edge of the lens and initially not cause any symptoms.

People who have small cataracts can often see well enough around the cloudy areas to manage normally. Other people, however, find that they are unable to read, drive or live independently because of the resulting loss of vision. A cataract may cause one or a combination of the following symptoms.

Mistiness or blurring of vision

This usually comes on gradually, although a posterior subcapsular cataract can cause deterioration in your vision over a few weeks or months. The mistiness is

Normal healthy eye

This illustration shows the detail of the front section of the eye.

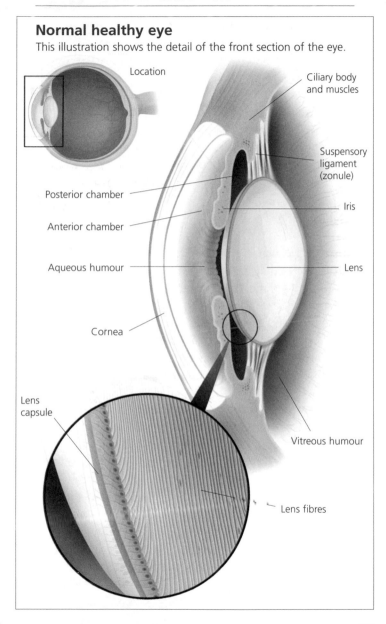

Location

Ciliary body and muscles

Suspensory ligament (zonule)

Posterior chamber

Iris

Anterior chamber

Aqueous humour

Lens

Cornea

Lens capsule

Vitreous humour

Lens fibres

usually spread throughout your field of vision and affects both distance and reading vision. Both of your eyes can be affected, although one is usually worse than the other.

Extreme sensitivity to bright light

Dazzling can result from bright sunlight, or at night from car headlights. It can be quite disabling but is helped by wearing dark glasses. However, wearing dark glasses will also reduce the amount of light getting into the eye, therefore making your overall level of vision slightly worse.

Reduced colour vision

This is particularly common with nuclear sclerotic cataracts. As the cataracts mature and become more yellow or brown, they tend to cut out light, particularly at the blue end of the colour spectrum, making colours appear much duller. After cataract surgery, people are often amazed to find how bright colours can be – for example, in the garden or on home furnishings.

Ghosting of images or double vision

This is most commonly found in people with cortical cataracts. It usually occurs with each eye separately and therefore is present even with one eye closed. It is often only a minor irritant and does not significantly affect most people with cataracts. Ghosting of the images consists of appreciation of a vague second image of an object that overlaps the main image. This contrasts with frank, or distinct, double vision where two strong images of an object are seen separately.

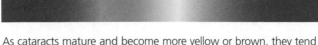

As cataracts mature and become more yellow or brown, they tend to cut out light, particularly at the blue end of the spectrum.

A shadow in the field of vision

This symptom is occasionally experienced by people with cataracts (particularly if they have the posterior subcapsular variety). It can also be the result of retinal disease but a visit to your optometrist should be able to identify the cause.

Making a diagnosis

If your vision is blurred or you have any of the signs or symptoms described, it is advisable to seek help early on in order to establish a definite diagnosis. These symptoms can occasionally be caused by other eye conditions. Initially, make an appointment to see your own optometrist or doctor. He or she will be able to advise you on the likely cause of your symptoms and can, if necessary, refer you to an ophthalmologist or ophthalmic surgeon at your local hospital for a more comprehensive eye examination.

A hospital eye specialist will identify the kind of cataract that you have. You will have a sight test and a full eye examination using a specialist slit-lamp microscope (see page 51). This examination involves dilating the pupils with drops, which will make the vision blurred for 8 to 10 hours afterwards and you will be unable to drive for this period.

When do cataracts need treatment?

Many people with mild cataracts carry on without difficulty. These people do not require any treatment until their vision deteriorates sufficiently to begin to affect their everyday life. Cataracts no longer have to become severe or very dense before surgery can be carried out. In fact, a dense cataract can be more difficult to operate on with the newer small-incision surgery than less advanced cases.

Seek advice early

In many eye units in the UK, there is still a significant waiting list for cataract surgery. Therefore, an early diagnosis can help prevent a severe loss of vision before cataract surgery can be carried out. If cataracts are left untreated for many years, they may eventually become mature, with the entire lens becoming milky white. Cataracts rarely develop to this maturity in developed countries, although they still commonly occur in developing countries where cataract surgery is not so readily available.

It is especially important to seek early advice if you are suffering from other disabilities, such as hearing loss or poor mobility, because a combination of these with reduced vision can increase the risk of accidents.

Is treatment safe?

Cataract surgery in developed countries such as Britain is now a relatively safe procedure and is successful in the great majority of cases. However, if other eye diseases (such as macular degeneration) also affect your vision, cataract surgery may not necessarily restore your vision completely. Cataract surgery is discussed in more detail in the next chapter.

Driving and cataracts

Your ability to drive is often affected early on by cataracts, as a result of both misting of the vision and dazzle from car headlights, street lighting or bright sunshine.

Your visual acuity has to be reduced from normal only by about 20 per cent to be below the legal limits required in the UK for driving a private motor vehicle. If you are unsure, ask your optometrist or doctor for advice.

KEY POINTS

■ If you have a cataract, the lens of your eye is cloudy rather than clear

■ Cataracts have many causes, but most are the result of ageing

■ Cataracts can cause blurred vision, dazzle, reduced colour vision, double vision and shadows in your vision

■ Cataract surgery is usually very successful and is a relatively safe procedure

Cataract surgery

Types of surgery

If you have a cataract, you may need surgery to improve the sight in your affected eye. This involves removing the lens containing the cataract from your eye and usually replacing it with an artificial lens (called an intraocular lens implant).The first lens implant in the world was carried out at St Thomas' Hospital in London in 1949 by a British ophthalmic surgeon called Sir Harold Ridley.

Many people think that cataract surgery is carried out with a laser, but this is not actually the case. There are four well-recognised forms of cataract surgery carried out in the world today: phacoemulsification, small incision non-phacoemulsification cataract surgery (SICS), extracapsular cataract surgery and intracapsular cataract surgery. All units in the UK have, since the 1990s, taken up the technique of phacoemulsification, as it requires only a small incision and the patient's sight recovers quickly after surgery.

Phacoemulsification

This is the most modern form of cataract surgery and is the operation of choice in most developed countries. The surgical incision used is very small – only 2.2 to 6 mm long. The small incision has many advantages: the wound heals quickly; visual rehabilitation is complete within three to four weeks; and often no stitches (sutures) are required.

Another significant advantage of this type of surgery is the fact that the wound causes little or no postoperative astigmatism (see 'Common sight problems', page 23). Phacoemulsification enables the surgeon to have more control over the pressure within the eye during the operation, preventing collapse of the eye and reducing the risk of operative complications. Phacoemulsification is suitable for most cataracts, although mature or hard cataractous lenses can be more difficult to remove using this technique.

The operation

At the beginning of the operation, the surgeon makes a small incision in the cornea, through which small instruments are inserted. Initially he or she creates a circular window in the front part of the lens capsule.

An ultrasonic probe is then introduced into the eye to divide and emulsify (soften and liquefy) the cataractous nucleus of the lens, which can then be sucked out through a small tube. The soft outer cortical lens matter is then removed using suction and, in most cases, a prosthetic (artificial) lens implant is introduced into the eye and placed within the remaining capsular bag, thus ensuring that the implant is fixed in the lens' natural position in the eye.

What happens during phacoemulsification?

Phacoemulsification is the most modern form of cataract surgery.

First stage
A small incision is made in the cornea and a tiny circular window in the front of the lens capsule

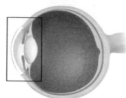

Location

Small incision in the cornea

Circular incision in the lens capsule

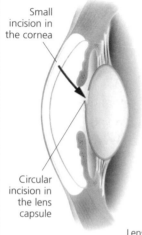

Second stage
An ultrasonic probe is introduced into the eye to soften the lens nucleus, so that it can be sucked out through a tube

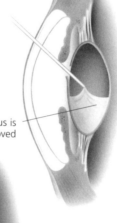

Lens nucleus is removed

Remaining lens capsule

Prosthetic lens is implanted

Third stage
An artificial lens implant is placed in the eye within the remaining capsular bag

Artificial lenses

There are many types of prosthetic lens and, until recently, Perspex lenses were the most common variety. These days, many surgeons prefer to use acrylic or silicone lens implants. This is because these implants can be folded, making it easier to insert them into the eye through the tiny incision. The implant then unfolds inside the eye to sit within the capsular bag. It is supported by the curved arms of the lens implant, known as 'haptics'.

New intraocular lenses are being developed that may achieve some 'accommodation', that is the ability to alter the focus from a distant to a near object. These lenses are not widely used and require long-term evaluation. Ask your consultant eye surgeon about the types of implants that he or she plans to use.

After cataract surgery by phacoemulsification, your normal vision will have substantially returned within a week, although it usually takes three to four weeks before full rehabilitation occurs and new glasses can be prescribed (if they are necessary).

Small incision non-phacoemulsification cataract surgery (SICS)

This form of surgery is not used in the UK but is increasingly being performed in developing countries. It does not require the expensive and sophisticated machinery used in phacoemulsification but still uses a fairly small incision (five to six millimetres) and is carried out using an operating microscope. In skilled hands the results are good.

Extracapsular cataract surgery

This form of cataract surgery has been used widely

What happens during extracapsular surgery?

This method is still used when the affected lens is too difficult to remove by phacoemulsification.

Location

First stage
An incision is made in the cornea and a window cut in the front of the lens capsule, through which the nucleus can be removed.

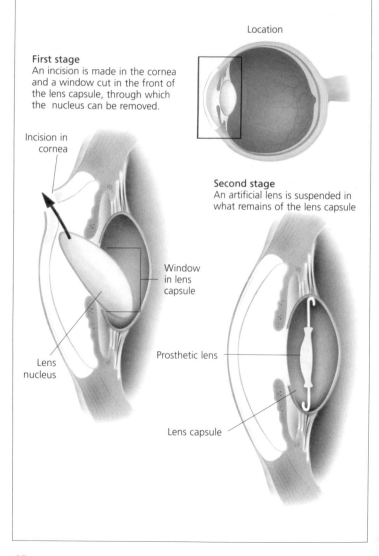

Incision in cornea

Window in lens capsule

Lens nucleus

Second stage
An artificial lens is suspended in what remains of the lens capsule

Prosthetic lens

Lens capsule

throughout the world since the 1960s and is still practised in many countries. It is used occasionally in developed countries when the affected lens is deemed too difficult to remove by phacoemulsification, for example if the lens is particularly hard. It is an effective form of cataract surgery but involves making a larger incision than for phacoemulsification. The wound is 10 to 15 mm long and requires 5 or 6 stitches to close it after the removal of the lens. Surgically induced astigmatism can result, however, requiring removal of the stitches and/or a change of prescription for your glasses. Visual rehabilitation is slower than after phacoemulsification – it may take three months. However, extracapsular cataract surgery is suitable for all kinds of cataractous lenses, even those that are mature or hard in texture.

The operation

During extracapsular surgery, a window is cut in the front surface of the lens capsule. Through this hole the centrally situated nucleus is removed in one piece from the eye. The surrounding cortical material is then vacuumed out using a special suction instrument. In most cases, a prosthetic lens implant is then inserted into the resulting space in the capsular bag. The capsular bag holds the lens implant in the position within the eye normally occupied by the natural lens.

Intracapsular cataract surgery

This operation is now seldom carried out in developed countries, but it may still be necessary in certain circumstances, for instance when the zonules supporting the lens are too weak. Intracapsular surgery involves the removal of the entire lens, including the outer

What happens during intracapsular surgery?

This operation requires a larger incision than other types of cataract surgery and the entire lens is removed.

Location

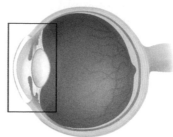

First stage
An incision is made in the cornea, large enough for the surgeon to remove the entire lens

Incision in cornea

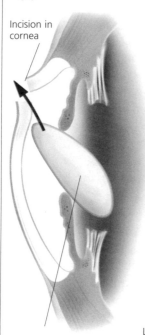

Second stage
A new artificial lens is placed across the front of the iris, over the pupil

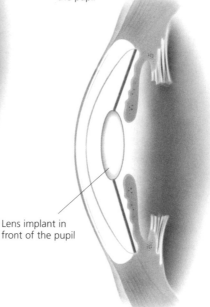

Entire lens is removed

Lens implant in front of the pupil

capsule, which is left in place in phacoemulsification and extracapsular cataract surgery. Great care is taken to ensure that the front face of the vitreous humour (which lies behind the lens) remains intact so that the vitreous and aqueous humour do not mix, because this can lead to complications such as retinal tears and detachments. Lens implantation is still possible but the implant has to be placed in front of the iris and spans the pupil. If a lens is not implanted vision can be corrected by glasses but these are very thick and powerful and do not restore visual function perfectly. In a similar fashion to extracapsular surgery, a relatively large incision is needed together with five or more stitches. Intracapsular surgery is still carried out in developing countries because the operation is quick and simple, allowing many people to be operated on by a single surgeon in one day. However, the results of intracapsular cataract surgery are not as good as the other two methods described, which is why it has fallen out of favour in most developed countries.

Benefits and risks of cataract surgery

As with all forms of surgery, it is important to ensure that the benefits of surgery outweigh the potential risks. If the cataract interferes with sight so much that the quality of vision is significantly reduced, then the benefits of cataract surgery can be very great.

The risks of surgery, particularly phacoemulsification and extracapsular cataract surgery, are small and about 95 per cent of patients have trouble-free surgery and a successful visual outcome.

For the remaining five per cent, complications may occur, but these are frequently minor in nature and usually settle in the first few weeks after surgery.

Significant sight-threatening complications, such as infection inside the eye, can occur in 1 in 400 to 1 in 1,000 cases. It is advisable to consult your ophthalmic surgeon to discuss the pros and cons of surgery so that a balanced decision can be reached.

Assessment for surgery

Having been diagnosed with a cataract and referred to an ophthalmic surgeon, he or she will carry out a comprehensive examination of your eyes. Your pupils will be dilated to allow the cataract to be properly assessed and the retina to be examined to ensure that there are no retinal problems that might contribute to the reduction in your vision.

If your pupils do have to be dilated this will blur your vision and preclude driving for 8 to 10 hours.

Some people with cataracts also have coexisting macular disease (see page 98), which may prevent the return of perfect vision even after the cataract has been removed. Nevertheless, in many cases, the removal of the cataract can improve the vision substantially and is still worthwhile. Your ophthalmic surgeon will be able to advise you.

Biometry testing

Once surgery has been decided on, the surgeon will need to carry out a number of tests. These will enable him or her to decide the strength of the artificial intraocular lens that will be implanted into your eye.

These tests are straightforward and painless, and involve measuring the curvature of the front surface of your cornea and the length of your eye (using an ultrasonic or infrared measure). This process is called

Slit-lamp examination

A slit-lamp produces a narrow beam of intense light that allows examination of the structures of the eye. The pupils must be fully dilated with eyedrops if the retina is to be thoroughly examined.

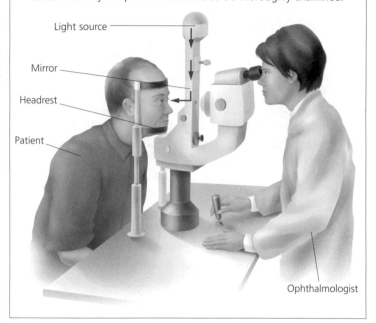

Light source

Mirror

Headrest

Patient

Ophthalmologist

'biometry' and is usually carried out a day or two before the operation.

Selecting the lens

The power of the intraocular lens implant selected is the one that is most appropriate to your current glasses prescription and desired postoperative refraction (power of the glasses). By implanting an artificial lens, the surgeon can significantly reduce, or even eliminate, long-sightedness or short-sightedness in people who have previously had to wear strong glasses. Your surgeon will discuss the postoperative refraction that you wish to have and will aim to achieve this by selecting an appropriate lens implant power.

The choice of the postoperative refraction will also be dictated by the power of the spectacle lens for your other eye because it is important not to create an imbalance between the two eyes by having one spectacle lens much stronger than the other one. This is called 'anisometropia'.

In addition, some people who have been short-sighted (myopic) all their lives prefer to stay short-sighted, although most prefer to take the opportunity to eliminate or reduce their short-sightedness. If the refraction is set to be neutral for distance, then glasses will still be needed for reading.

As we get older the natural lens inside the eye becomes less malleable and will therefore not change shape or 'accommodate' for reading, which is why people need reading glasses in middle age. Therefore replacing a natural lens with a lens implant that has a fixed focus does not create problems for older patients. There have been a number of trials of multifocal and 'accommodating' intraocular lenses, but the latter variety has not yet proved popular because of the difficulty of achieving good vision for both distance and near vision.

Multifocal lens implants are increasingly being offered to patients, although not on the NHS. These lens implants can give vision for both reading vision and distance vision but spectacles may also be needed. They are not suitable for all patients and the lens implants need to be carefully centred. If you are considering multifocal lens implants, discuss the pros and cons with your eye surgeon.

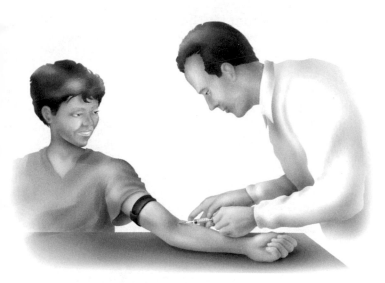

It may be necessary for you to have blood taken for tests.

Other preoperative checks

Your consultant will also check for any possible sources of infection from your eyelids (blepharitis), conjunctiva (conjunctivitis) or elsewhere in the body, such as urinary infections or leg ulcers. These sources of infection need to be treated with antibiotics before surgery in order to reduce the risk of infectious contamination during the operation.

The consultant will also carry out a general assessment of your eye and will check the state of the retina. Your anaesthetist will assess your general health and appropriateness for a local or general anaesthetic.

Many parts of the preoperative assessment may be carried out by a suitably trained nurse. It may be necessary for you to have blood taken for tests and to have an electrocardiogram (ECG), especially if a general

Electrocardiogram (ECG)

Before general anaesthesia, an electrocardiogram (ECG) is often required to check and record the electrical activity of your heart.

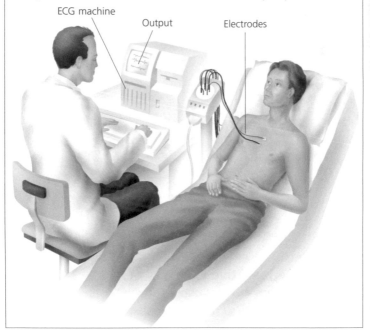

ECG machine

Output

Electrodes

anaesthetic is being considered. If you are allergic to any medications, drops or sticking plaster, it is important to tell your preoperative assessment nurse, surgeon and anaesthetist.

Medications that can affect your cataract surgery

Blood-thinning agents such as warfarin can increase the risk of bleeding during cataract surgery and the dose of warfarin may need to be altered before the operation. Certain medications that help urinary flow, for example tamsulosin hydrochloride, can alter the rigidity of the iris and cause difficulties during cataract surgery. It is important to give a full list of medications that you are using to the eye surgeon, anaesthetist and preoperative assessment nurse before your operation.

Day-case or inpatient surgery?

Cataract surgery is usually straightforward and should not cause you any constitutional upset. It can be carried out as a day case or as an inpatient (overnight stay). The decision about whether cataract surgery

Questions to ask your consultant

- How straightforward is this procedure?
- Do I have any other eye diseases that could affect the outcome of the operation?
- Do I have any other health problems that could complicate the operation?
- Will you be inserting an artificial lens and, if so, which type?
- Will I be able to have day-case surgery?
- Will I have a local or a general anaesthetic?
- What are my chances of having poorer vision after the operation or losing the sight in the eye?
- I am taking regular medications. Can I take them on the day of the operation, and if so when?
- Can I eat or drink before surgery. If not, when do I have to stop?
- How long will the healing process take?
- Will I have to wear glasses or contact lenses afterwards?
- Are there any activities that I should avoid after the operation?

should be carried out as a day case or an overnight stay will be made with your surgeon and anaesthetist.

Day-case surgery

Most people prefer day-case surgery. In this situation, you come in on the day of the operation a few hours before surgery, and can go home the same day after having been seen by the surgeon on his or her postoperative ward round. Your eye usually needs a postoperative check-up the next day at the hospital; this is carried out by your surgeon or a trained nurse, although in some centres they phone you at home to ask how you are getting on.

If day-case surgery is being considered, it is important that you are well with no serious conditions, such as angina or severe chest disease, and that you have home support available for the night after the operation, together with transport to and from the hospital. Although most day-case cataract surgery is carried out under a local anaesthetic, having a general anaesthetic does not preclude a day-case stay.

Overnight stays

If you have no home support, are infirm or have a significant medical condition, inpatient surgery will probably be more appropriate. You may come in the day before your operation or sometimes on the day itself and usually stay for one night afterwards.

The choice of anaesthetic

Cataract surgery can be carried out under either a local or a general anaesthetic. Most patients have a local anaesthetic, but the decision depends on your preference and the advice of your surgeon and the anaesthetist.

Local anaesthetic

If you have a local anaesthetic, it is given by an injection through either your conjunctiva or the skin beneath the eye, so that the anaesthetic bathes the area around the eye, and prevents it from feeling anything or moving during the operation. One or two injections may be necessary.

Under some circumstances, the local anaesthetic may also prevent your eye seeing anything during surgery. Even if this is not the case, most patients are aware of only vague shadows in their field of view during the operation. The local anaesthetic injection wears off three to five hours after the operation.

Some surgeons carry out cataract surgery using topical anaesthesia. This involves using anaesthetic drops on your eye, which prevent feeling but allow the eye to move normally. This approach avoids an injection and is preferred by some people. Additional anaesthesia can be administered during the operation if necessary.

You may be asked not to eat for four to five hours before your operation and not to drink for two hours, but it is important to find out from your anaesthetist and surgeon the particular protocol that they adopt. If you are on any medication, ask when you should take them. Premedications (such as sedatives or tranquillisers) are not usually necessary and may not be desirable because they may cause you to fall asleep and wake with a start during surgery.

General anaesthetic

If you have a general anaesthetic, you may be given premedication an hour or so before surgery and you will be unconscious throughout the operation. General anaesthesia for cataract surgery does not have to be particularly deep, and the postoperative recovery period is usually quick, with little nausea or after-effect.

You will be asked to have nothing to eat or drink for five or more hours before the operation. If you are taking medicines for heart disease or high blood pressure, it is important that you take them on the day of your operation; ask your surgeon or anaesthetist about timing.

The operation

During the hour before surgery, one of the nurses on the ward will administer drops into your eye to dilate (widen) the pupil. This is to enable the surgeon to remove the cataractous lens through the dilated pupil. If you are having your operation under a local anaesthetic, it is important to wear your hearing aid (if you have one) but you do not need to remove any dentures.

Modern cataract surgery usually takes half an hour or less. During the operation, you will be lying flat on the operating table and the position of the table can be altered to make you more comfortable. It is important that you remain calm and still during the procedure. A paper or cloth drape is placed over your head, face and chest. This is held away from your nose and mouth, and fresh air and oxygen are fed in under the drape so that you can breathe comfortably.

If you are having a local anaesthetic, a nurse will hold your hand throughout the operation. This is a natural source of comfort, but also acts as a form of communication between you and your surgeon. If you wish to speak or move, then squeezing the nurse's hand twice will enable the nurse to tell your surgeon to pause and find out what you wish to say.

The eyelids of the eye being operated upon will be held open during the operation; you therefore do not need to be concerned about blinking. You can also close the other eye.

To remove the cataractous lens, the surgeon will use a surgical microscope that incorporates a bright light that shines onto your eye but does not usually cause any discomfort. At the end of the operation, the surgeon will administer antibiotics and/or sterilising drops to your eye, then cover the eye with a protective pad or shield secured with special tape.

Postoperative recovery and treatment

Immediately after the operation, you will be taken to the recovery bay before going back to the ward. If a local anaesthetic was used, you may be able simply to go straight back to the ward in a wheelchair or sit in an armchair in the recovery area. After recovery, you can have a drink and something to eat and, if you are being treated as a day case, you can go home.

Immediate aftercare

Sometimes, you will be given tablets to prevent a pressure rise in your eye during the immediate postoperative period. The eye shield or pad will remain in place until your eye has been checked by the surgeon or nurse the next day. Your level of vision is usually measured the day after the operation, and your vision may be improved but not necessarily very sharp at this stage. Your vision usually recovers quickly during the first few days after surgery. Sometimes patients do not have to come back to the hospital the day after surgery. Instead, they are telephoned by a specialist nurse to ensure that the eye is settling satisfactorily and to give advice.

After the surgery there may be some discomfort in the eye but there is not normally any significant pain. Simple pain relief tablets may be taken if the eye is uncomfortable. If there is significant pain then you should tell the nursing staff on the ward or telephone the hospital if you are already at home.

If you have had a local anaesthetic you may experience some double vision as the anaesthetic wears off but this usually resolves within six to eight hours of the operation. Your eye may be light sensitive for a few days and it is wise to have a pair of dark glasses.

Ongoing care

Your nurse will advise you about how to care for the eye that has been operated on. Some additional advice is set out below.

Eye drops

Most people are given antibiotic and anti-inflammatory drops to put in the eye for a few weeks after the operation. These drops reduce eye inflammation and prevent infection. Detailed instructions will be given to you before discharge. Most people are able to apply these drops themselves, but if you find it difficult a relative or district nurse can help.

Outpatient appointment

You will usually be seen as an outpatient once or twice after the operation, with the final check being made about six weeks after cataract surgery. If your eye aches or your vision deteriorates, this may be a sign of a potential problem with your eye; you should quickly contact the eye ward or your surgeon for advice.

Glasses

Immediately after your operation, your sight may be blurred. You can wear your present glasses (or dark glasses) if they help; however, you will probably need new glasses three to four weeks after surgery. You will be asked to go to your optometrist for these.

If you had stitches

Occasionally you require stitches for your eye wound during surgery. These are commonly made of nylon and are usually inert (non-reactive). They are often removed in the first few months after the operation.

The removal of the stitches is very straightforward and is carried out as an outpatient procedure using anaesthetic drops. If the stitches are not removed, sometimes months or years after the operation, the stitches can break causing a foreign body sensation in the eye. If this happens, the broken stitch or stitches can be removed by an eye surgeon using an examining microscope – this is also an outpatient procedure carried out under local anaesthetic drops.

Resuming day-to-day activities

You should avoid heavy lifting and straining for about four weeks after the operation, but otherwise you can carry on as normal. Most people can return to work after two weeks. You may bend normally but take care not to knock your eye.

Driving

It is best to avoid driving, at least until after your first outpatient visit, when you can ask the surgeon if your vision is good enough.

Protecting your eye at night

Most surgeons will ask you to wear your protective eye shield over the eye for the first week after surgery.

If you have had a stitch in the wound of your eye, you may not need to wear the shield after the first night.

Bathing and hairwashing

For the first week, avoid getting your eye wet and avoid rubbing, touching or pressing on it. You may wash your hair or go to the hairdresser but you should wear your protective eye shield for this.

Possible complications

Complications during and after cataract surgery are rare, and 95 per cent of patients have trouble-free operations.

During surgery

In a small number of cases (usually two per cent or less), the membrane within the eye (the posterior capsule) may break during the operation, allowing the vitreous humour (the jelly within the back part of the eye) to come forward. Usually it is straightforward to remove the vitreous humour surgically during the cataract operation so that a lens implant can be successfully inserted into the eye and the vision restored. If the vitreous humour is removed it is replaced by other inert fluid.

After surgery

Bleeding

Occasionally, there is some bleeding beneath the surface of your eye (subconjunctival haemorrhage) and, although this looks dramatic, it usually clears up without difficulty within a week or two and does not affect the outcome of the operation.

Inflammation

In the first few days after the operation, your eye can become inflamed (called uveitis or iritis). This generally clears up when treated with anti-inflammatory drops.

'Water logging'

Another possible complication is the onset of 'water logging' at the central part of the retina (macular oedema). This consists of an accumulation of fluid within the layers of the retina at the macula and is more common if the posterior capsule ruptures during the operation. This can affect your detailed vision but once again it frequently clears up after a few weeks or months.

Infection

A rare but serious complication can occur if the inside of the operated eye becomes infected (endophthalmitis). This occurs in between 1 in 400 and 1 in 1,000 patients. It usually occurs within a few days of the operation and is characterised by the onset of severe aching in, and/or around, the eye and is associated with blurring of the vision.

If these symptoms do occur, it is important to contact your surgeon or the eye ward immediately for advice. If caught early enough, intensive treatment with antibiotics can clear up the infection and give a good visual outcome.

Posterior capsule opacification

In some cases, the membrane that lies behind the lens implant (the posterior capsule) may become cloudy (opaque) after the operation. If this happens, it occurs months or years after surgery, and generally takes at least six months to appear.

The likelihood of this happening depends on a number of factors, including your age and the type of lens implant used. It is more common in young people and is less common with some lens designs and materials than others. There are many different kinds of implants used and if you are concerned you should discuss the issue with your surgeon. Opacification of the posterior capsule results in a misting of the vision, similar to the effect of the original cataract.

Fortunately it is easily treated as an outpatient procedure using a laser mounted on an examination microscope. You may need local anaesthetic drops and a contact lens and the procedure takes about 10 minutes.

After the laser treatment, your vision will be restored and further clouding of the posterior capsule does not usually occur. The procedure is straightforward and is easily tolerated even by elderly or infirm people. Complications are rare, although there is a small increase in the risk of developing a retinal tear, detachment or cystoid macular oedema.

Complications are not common

I have described most of the complications that can occur with cataract surgery. Reading about these complications could unnerve you, so remember that for the vast majority of people cataract surgery is straightforward and leads to an excellent visual result.

Glasses after cataract surgery

If the cataract has been removed using the phacoemulsification technique, your eye will be sufficiently well healed three to six weeks after surgery to enable you to have new glasses if necessary.

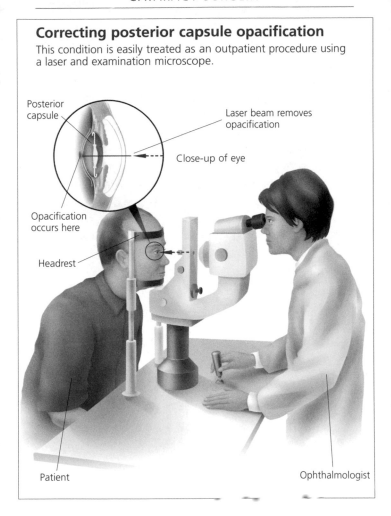

Correcting posterior capsule opacification

This condition is easily treated as an outpatient procedure using a laser and examination microscope.

Posterior capsule

Laser beam removes opacification

Close-up of eye

Opacification occurs here

Headrest

Patient

Ophthalmologist

If extracapsular surgery has been carried out, you must wait for two to three months. This is because the wound is much larger and so takes longer to heal.

The prosthetic lens implant cannot change its power in the way that a natural lens can. You therefore usually need glasses for reading and fine tuning of the distance vision. Varifocal lenses or bifocal lenses may be appropriate; ask your optometrist.

During your preoperative assessment and biometry, your eye surgeon will have selected a lens implant to suit your needs. This may mean that the glasses you need now will be much less powerful than those used before or you may not need them for distance vision.

Your surgeon will either refract your eye (assess any optical errors) himself or give you a letter to take to your optometrist for refraction and new glasses. There may be some changes in your prescription over the first few months after surgery, so you should visit your optometrist for a further check-up about six months after the operation.

KEY POINTS

■ Cataract surgery involves removing the cloudy lens and replacing it with an implant

■ Phacoemulsification is the most common type of cataract surgery. It uses a very small incision and most patients recover their vision very quickly

■ Surgery can be a day-case or inpatient procedure and may be performed under a local or general anaesthetic

■ Most patients return to their normal routine quickly, and complications are rare

Glaucoma

Is glaucoma serious?

Glaucoma is a leading cause of blindness in the UK. It tends to affect people aged over 40 and, in most cases, there are no warning symptoms until the late stages. Damage that has occurred before diagnosis cannot be reversed. However, blindness can be prevented if the condition is diagnosed and treated early on. For this reason, it is essential that you have regular eye examinations.

If you have been diagnosed with glaucoma, ask your ophthalmologist to explain the condition and treatment to you, and outline the possible effects of the condition in the future.

What is glaucoma?

The term 'glaucoma' is used to describe a group of eye conditions characterised by damage to the optic nerve within the eye, resulting in gradual loss of your peripheral vision (vision at the sides of your field of vision). This process is generally very gradual and is usually associated with a higher than normal pressure within your eye (known as intraocular pressure or IOP). The upper limit of normal pressure is defined as 21 millimetres of mercury (21 mmHg). If the intraocular pressure is too high, the optic nerve can be damaged.

Types of glaucoma

There are two main types of glaucoma:

1 open-angle glaucoma
2 angle-closure glaucoma.

Open-angle glaucoma comes on gradually (a long-term, or chronic, condition) and there are no warning symptoms until there has been considerable damage to the optic nerve and associated loss of the visual field.

Angle-closure glaucoma is much more sudden in onset (an acute condition) and produces severe symptoms.

The cause of glaucoma

To understand the difference between these two forms of glaucoma, you need to know about the production and drainage of fluid in the front chamber of the eye. This fluid (aqueous humour) is continuously produced within the eye by the ciliary body, which lies in the midpoint of the eye close to the lens. Normally, the fluid passes forwards through the pupil and drains away into the bloodstream.

One source of drainage is called the trabecular meshwork, which is responsible for most of the fluid outflow, and the other is the uveoscleral pathway. The trabecular meshwork is found in the point, or 'angle', where the iris meets the cornea (called the drainage angle).

Normally, the amount of fluid produced is the same as the amount of fluid draining out. However, if the fluid cannot escape, or too much is produced, the pressure within the eye will rise.

Open-angle glaucoma

In this form of glaucoma, the drainage angle is open but it does not allow enough fluid to drain away from within the eye, because either the drainage angle is partially blocked or the eye produces too much aqueous humour. So the fluid builds up and causes a rise in the pressure within the eye. This pressure rise is usually slow and painless.

Angle-closure glaucoma

In this form, the drainage angle becomes closed by the iris and the fluid is unable to drain from the eye. This usually happens quite quickly and the pressure rise is much greater than that of open-angle glaucoma. It is usually accompanied by severe symptoms such as marked aching in the eye and blurring. These symptoms are described in more detail on page 83. Angle-closure glaucoma, also known as closed-angle glaucoma, is a medical emergency.

Ocular hypertension and glaucoma

Some people have an open drainage angle but also have a moderate rise in intraocular pressure with no other signs of open-angle glaucoma (optic nerve damage or visual field loss). In some people, their intraocular pressure is higher than 21 mmHg but this is still normal for them, whereas, in others, pressures of over 21 mmHg may be an early sign of glaucoma. If someone has raised intraocular pressure without other signs of glaucoma, they are classed as having 'ocular hypertension'. These people do not require eye treatment unless they show the other signs of developing glaucoma or have predisposing factors such as a family history of glaucoma. They will, however, be monitored regularly to see if further signs develop.

Other forms of glaucoma

There are many different kinds of glaucoma other than those described here, but they are rare and do not merit detailed consideration here. So-called secondary glaucoma can occur as a result of other conditions within the eye such as inflammation (uveitis or iritis). Developmental glaucoma in babies is caused by a malformation in the eye of the fetus in the uterus and is very rare in the UK.

Open-angle glaucoma
Causes of open-angle glaucoma

The specific cause of open-angle glaucoma is unknown. However, it seems to be a combination of higher than normal pressure within the eye and a less effective blood supply to your optic nerve. The rise in intraocular pressure is thought to result from a reduced ability of the drainage angle to drain the fluid from within the eye.

There are a number of factors that increase the risk of a person developing open-angle glaucoma. It is not possible to prevent it from developing, but early diagnosis and careful treatment can help to halt or slow its progression. Most optometrists in the UK will routinely test for glaucoma and refer you to the hospital eye service if they are suspicious.

It is therefore wise to visit your optometrist at least once every two years for an eye test and more often if recommended. If you have a mother, father, sister, brother or child (known as a first-degree relative) with

Main forms of glaucoma

Glaucoma is usually associated with abnormally high pressure in the eye, commonly because the fluid bathing the front of the eye cannot escape. This can be because there is too much fluid, or because the drainage angle is partially blocked or closed. If the pressure remains high permanent damage to the optic nerve can occur.

Normal eye

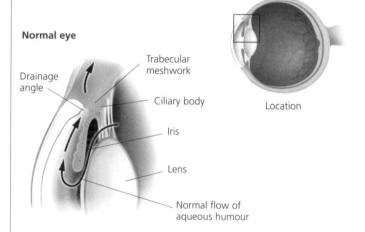

Drainage angle

Trabecular meshwork

Ciliary body

Iris

Lens

Normal flow of aqueous humour

Location

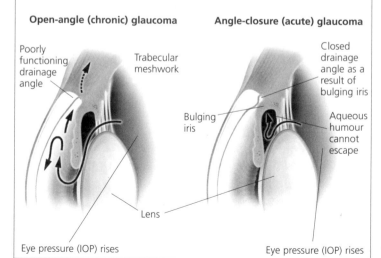

Open-angle (chronic) glaucoma

Poorly functioning drainage angle

Trabecular meshwork

Lens

Eye pressure (IOP) rises

Angle-closure (acute) glaucoma

Closed drainage angle as a result of bulging iris

Bulging iris

Aqueous humour cannot escape

Eye pressure (IOP) rises

the condition, you should have an annual check-up and you will not be charged for it. The following are the main risk factors for open-angle glaucoma.

Older age
Open-angle glaucoma is much more common with increasing age. It is rare below the age of 40 but affects 1 per cent of the population aged 40 and above, and 5 per cent of people over the age of 65.

Family history
If you have a first-degree relative with glaucoma, there is an increased risk of you developing the condition. This risk has not been accurately defined, but is in the region of one in five. Everyone who has a first-degree relative with glaucoma should have their intraocular pressure monitored annually.

Short-sightedness (myopia)
People who are short-sighted are more likely to develop glaucoma than others.

Ethnic origin
People of African origin have a greater risk of developing open-angle glaucoma. The condition may develop at a younger age than in other people.

Symptoms of open-angle glaucoma
If you have open-angle glaucoma, you may not actually notice any symptoms, unless the condition is very advanced, in which case you may notice some loss of peripheral (side) vision. The condition is entirely painless and your central vision is generally not affected until the disease is at an advanced stage.

Damage that has already been done to the retinal nerve fibres and optic nerve by the time the glaucoma is diagnosed cannot be reversed. However, with early diagnosis and careful treatment, the damage can usually be restricted and the progression of the disease slowed down or even halted. If untreated, chronic open-angle glaucoma can eventually lead to a severe loss of vision or even blindness. Therefore early diagnosis and treatment are vital.

Making a diagnosis

The diagnosis of open-angle glaucoma is commonly made by an ophthalmologist after referral by an optometrist or your doctor and is based on three main factors:

1 Raised pressure within the eye (intraocular pressure) – usually greater than 21 mmHg.
2 Characteristic loss of visual field, although you may not notice this because it is so gradual.
3 Cupping of the optic nerve within the eye (where the optic nerve head becomes concave as a result of the loss of nerve fibres within it).

The three tests for glaucoma are:

1 optic nerve assessment
2 tonometry
3 perimetry.

Optic nerve head assessment

The retina and optic nerve are examined by shining a light from a special instrument (ophthalmoscope) into your eye or examining the eye with a special lens in conjunction with a biomicroscope (a slit-lamp). Any cupping and paleness of the optic nerve head in the eye are characteristic signs of glaucoma.

Ophthalmoscope

An ophthalmoscope is used to examine the retina and optic nerve.

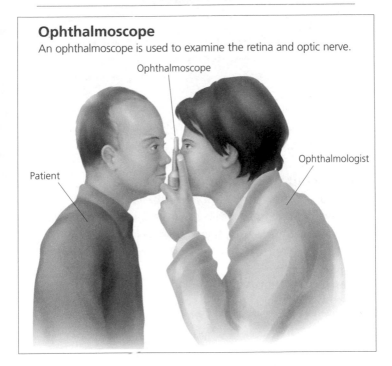

Ophthalmoscope

Ophthalmologist

Patient

Some eye units are now assessing the optic nerve head using a 'scanning laser ophthalmoscope', which creates a contour map of the optic nerve. This is simple and painless to perform.

Tonometry

Intraocular pressure is measured using a special instrument called a tonometer. In hospital eye departments this involves the application of anaesthetic drops. It is a quick simple procedure and the specialist looks into your eye with a slit-lamp bio-microscope. Many optometrists use a different method of measuring the pressure, directing a puff of air at the eye, which is less accurate.

Perimetry

Your visual field is examined to establish any loss in your peripheral vision using a perimeter. You sit with your chin on a rest looking straight at a small target. Spots of light of varying intensity are presented in the periphery (edge) of your visual field and you will be asked to press a buzzer when the spot is seen. The procedure takes about five minutes for each eye.

Treatment of open-angle glaucoma

The aim of treatment for long-term glaucoma is to reduce the pressure within the eye. This is frequently achieved with eye drops and, occasionally, tablets. If this fails, your ophthalmologist may suggest either

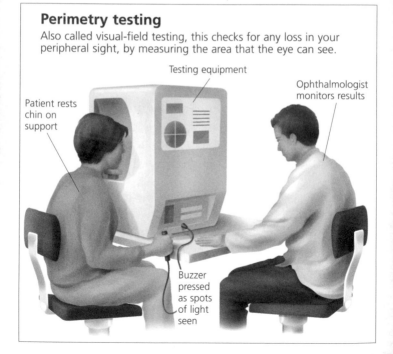

Perimetry testing

Also called visual-field testing, this checks for any loss in your peripheral sight, by measuring the area that the eye can see.

Testing equipment

Ophthalmologist monitors results

Patient rests chin on support

Buzzer pressed as spots of light seen

laser treatment or an operation called a trabeculectomy to improve drainage from the eye (see page 88).

Medication with eye drops

There are many different kinds of drops that can be used. Generally one type of drop will be tried initially and, if this does not lower the pressure sufficiently, further drops may be added.

Please note that the proper (or generic) names are used here to describe drops and other medications. Most medications are also known by their commercial (proprietary or brand) names, which are different from the proper names. Please ask your chemist if in doubt.

There can be side effects from the drops, although these are not usually serious. However, you should read the instruction leaflet.

If you have asthma or other chest problems or vascular or heart disease, you must tell your specialist as not all drops will be suitable. Some of the drops are believed to increase the blood supply to the optic nerve within your eye as well as lowering the pressure. The drops used for chronic open-angle glaucoma include the following groups.

Prostaglandins

These are hormone-like substances that keep your blood vessels dilated (widened) so that more fluid can flow through them. Examples used to treat glaucoma are latanoprost, travoprost and bimatoprost. They lower the pressure in the eye by increasing the outflow of the aqueous humour from the eye.

• Side effects: Prostaglandin drops appear to have few significant side effects on the body as a whole, but can cause the eyelashes to darken and lengthen and/or the iris to darken in colour.

Beta blockers

These drops are commonly used for glaucoma. They lower the pressure inside the eye, probably by reducing the production of aqueous fluid. The beta blockers for glaucoma are betaxolol, carteolol, levobunolol, metipranolol and timolol.

• Side effects: Beta blockers can trigger or exacerbate asthma or other forms of chest disease (such as chronic obstructive pulmonary disease) and are not advised for people with chest disease. More rarely beta-blocker eyedrops can slow the pulse and should be used with caution in patients who are using other heart medications (particularly beta-blocker tablets).

Furthermore, they are contraindicated in people with peripheral blood vessel disease causing cold hands and feet. They can also sometimes make the eyes feel dry and have been reported to cause sleepiness and lethargy.

Miotics

These drops contract the iris muscles and constrict the pupil. This pulls the iris away from the trabecular meshwork and allows the fluid to drain away more readily. The drugs used are carbachol and pilocarpine.

• Side effects: As miotics affect the pupil and the accommodation of the lens, they can interfere with reading vision and also make distance vision blurred.

They can also cause the eye to ache for 20 to 30 minutes after administration. These side effects often fade with continuing use. Miotic drops can make it more difficult for you to see in the dark because of the constriction of the pupil and, over a long period of time, can predispose to the development of cataracts.

Miotics are not used very frequently nowadays in the treatment of open-angle glaucoma, although they are one of the preferred treatments for angle-closure glaucoma (see pages 84–5).

Sympathomimetics

These drugs are believed to act by reducing the production of aqueous humour and by increasing the outflow through the trabecular meshwork. They are called adrenaline (epinephrine) and dipivefrine.

• Side effects: These drops tend to cause the superficial blood vessels of the eye to dilate, making the eye look red. Over a long period of time they have also been known to cause scarring beneath the conjunctiva.

Carbonic anhydrase inhibitors

These drops reduce the production of aqueous humour by the ciliary body. They are called brinzolamide and dorzolamide. Carbonic anhydrase inhibitors are also available in tablet form (as acetazolamide) and these act by reducing the fluid levels in the body.

• Side effects: If used for long periods the tablet form can cause an imbalance in the salts of the body (potassium loss in particular), and blood tests need to be carried out two or three times a year to monitor levels. In addition, carbonic anhydrase inhibitors commonly cause tingling of the extremities (in particular the fingers and toes).

Alpha-2 agonists
These drugs, brimonidine and apraclonidine, reduce the production of the aqueous humour from the ciliary body.

• Side effects: In approximately 15 per cent of cases these drops can cause marked allergic reactions in the eyes and cause redness and discomfort. This reaction may not occur until six months after starting the drops.

Medication with tablets
If the glaucoma cannot be controlled with drops alone, short-term control can be achieved with tablets. The most notable of these is a carbonic anhydrase inhibitor (see page 81) called acetazolamide, which acts by powerfully reducing the amount of fluid (aqueous humour) produced within your eye, thereby lowering the pressure.

However, it has a number of side effects – for example, tingling in the fingers and toes – and can lead to a reduction in your body's potassium level. It is therefore generally used only for short periods unless under the close supervision of the ophthalmologist or your doctor. Blood tests will be needed two or three times a year to monitor potassium levels.

Long-term monitoring of open-angle glaucoma
Most people with glaucoma are reviewed by their ophthalmologist two or three times a year. At each consultation, your intraocular pressure will be measured and the condition of the optic nerve will be checked. Your specialist will look inside your eye with the help of a bright light from the biomicroscope and a special lens. In addition, your optic nerve may be assessed using the scanning laser ophthalmoscope.

Your visual field will be tested every year (possibly more frequently immediately after the diagnosis) and photographs may be taken of the optic nerve head for your medical records.

Angle-closure glaucoma
Causes of angle-closure glaucoma

Angle-closure glaucoma is acute, which means that it arises suddenly. It is more common in people who are very long-sighted (hypermetropic), and these people may have worn spectacles since childhood. The condition is more common in people over the age of 40 and affects more women than men.

There are a variety of prescribed medicines that can increase the risk of angle-closure glaucoma, especially major tranquillisers used in the treatment of depression and other psychiatric conditions. Your doctor will advise you about the medicines that can predispose to the development of acute angle-closure glaucoma. You should also read the manufacturer's leaflet that accompanies your medication to see whether it could trigger acute glaucoma.

Symptoms of angle-closure glaucoma

In marked contrast to the lack of symptoms in early open-angle glaucoma, angle-closure glaucoma usually has many symptoms. Early symptoms may consist of mild aching in one eye, associated with blurred vision, and sometimes seeing coloured rainbow effects around lights.

These symptoms are more common in dim light or darkness and often improve after a night's sleep. If you are suffering from these symptoms, a visit to your optometrist may be helpful so that your eye can be examined for any factors that predispose to the development of angle-closure glaucoma.

In a severe attack, the pressure increase in the eye can be great and occur over a few hours. The eye becomes very painful with a marked ache that may extend around the eye to the brow and temple. It usually affects only one eye at a time. The eye becomes red, and the vision deteriorates and is blurred. The affected person may also experience nausea and vomiting. If these symptoms occur, you need an urgent referral to the hospital eye service. You can get this through your doctor or an optometrist.

Making a diagnosis

Although this is a relatively unusual disease, a busy eye unit in the UK will see one or two cases of acute angle-closure glaucoma per week. The diagnosis is made on the symptoms described above, together with a markedly raised intraocular pressure measured using tonometry (see page 77). The diagnosis will be established in the hospital eye accident and emergency department, but your optometrist or doctor will probably have suspected it when he or she arranged your referral.

Treating angle-closure glaucoma

The high pressure in the eye can be readily treated with drops and medicines, which are administered initially in the accident and emergency department. The medicines most commonly used are pilocarpine drops (see 'Miotics', page 80) and acetazolamide – often given by injection into a vein.

In addition you will be given pain relief and treatment for nausea and vomiting if necessary. The intraocular pressure usually reduces within a few hours, but most people are admitted to hospital for their treatment and to monitor the pressure after this. Most patients stay in hospital for only a few days. Steroid or other anti-inflammatory drops to reduce the accompanying inflammation in the eye are also usually given.

Once the eye pressure is back to normal and the eye is less inflamed, laser treatment is given to prevent future attacks of angle-closure glaucoma. The laser is used to make a small hole in the peripheral part of the iris, to allow the fluid (aqueous humour) to drain away without having to pass through the pupil. This treatment is called a 'peripheral iridotomy'.

It is a simple procedure that is often carried out in the outpatient department. Anaesthetic drops will be put in your eye, and a contact lens will be placed on the eye to provide a magnified view of the iris. The laser treatment is delivered using a slit-lamp biomicroscope similar to the one used to examine your eye. Your unaffected eye may also be treated with a laser to prevent an acute attack in this eye too.

If diagnosed and treated early, acute angle-closure glaucoma does not lead to any significant damage to the vision, optic nerve or visual fields. The laser treatment usually prevents further attacks. Further substantive treatment is needed only in a minority of patients who suffer from recurrent pressure rises. This often involves a surgical procedure similar to that carried out for open-angle glaucoma (a trabeculectomy, see page 88).

Driving and glaucoma

To reach the legal requirements to drive in the UK, your visual fields must be substantially normal. If your visual field has been damaged by glaucoma of any

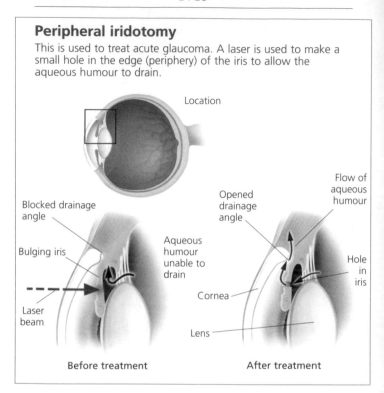

Peripheral iridotomy

This is used to treat acute glaucoma. A laser is used to make a small hole in the edge (periphery) of the iris to allow the aqueous humour to drain.

Location

Flow of aqueous humour

Opened drainage angle

Blocked drainage angle

Bulging iris

Aqueous humour unable to drain

Hole in iris

Cornea

Laser beam

Lens

Before treatment

After treatment

kind, you may fall below the required limits and your licence and insurance will not be valid. It is necessary for anyone who drives and has glaucoma to inform the Driver and Vehicle Licensing Agency (DVLA – see page 126) at Swansea. Your ophthalmologist or optometrist will then be asked to assess your visual function for driving and advise you accordingly.

KEY POINTS

■ Glaucoma involves damage to your optic nerve and is usually associated with raised pressure within your eye

■ Open-angle (chronic) glaucoma progresses slowly with few symptoms, and is most common with advancing age and in people with a family history of the condition

■ Open-angle glaucoma can be treated with eyedrops, tablets or, if these fail to work, surgery

■ Angle-closure (acute) glaucoma is sudden in onset and painful; it is treated as a medical emergency

■ Angle-closure glaucoma is treated with eyedrops and intravenous medicines, and later laser therapy to prevent future attacks

Surgery for open-angle glaucoma

Types of surgery

If you have chronic open-angle glaucoma, you may need to have surgery if the pressure in your eye cannot be controlled well enough with drops or other medicines.

The most common operation carried out in developed countries is called a trabeculectomy, although laser treatment may also be used. Your ophthalmologist will discuss which method of treatment is the best in your particular case. The operation can be carried out as a day case or with an overnight stay and, in a similar way to cataract surgery, it is often performed under a local anaesthetic.

Trabeculectomy

This operation is suitable for most varieties of open-angle glaucoma, but is used only when medication has failed. In trabeculectomy the surgeon forms a water blister (bleb) on the surface of the eye beneath the eyelid that allows fluid to drain from the eye in a controlled fashion. It is formed by drawing back a flap of the conjunctiva and then creating a trap door within the white scleral coat of the eye. Stitches are usually required but these biodegrade (dissolve) and disappear within a few weeks.

During the operation the surgeon makes a hole in the peripheral part of the iris, known as peripheral iridectomy, which allows the aqueous fluid (humour) to drain directly from the ciliary body to the front part of the inside of the eye, without having to pass through the pupil.

Trabeculectomy is usually very successful in controlling the pressure within the eye for a considerable period of time, sometimes many years.

Laser treatment

There are various forms of laser treatment available for open-angle glaucoma. Until recently one prevalent form of laser treatment was laser trabeculoplasty (LTP). This involves administering an argon gas laser under local anaesthetic drops, using a contact lens to view the drainage angle of the eye (the trabecular meshwork). The laser is applied to the trabecular meshwork and is said to work by opening up the pores of the meshwork, thereby allowing the aqueous fluid to drain more readily. This procedure is less popular now.

Diode laser

This form of laser treatment is more commonly used, but is reserved for patients whose intraocular pressure has not responded to either drops or trabeculectomy. This is carried out under a local anaesthetic, administered via an injection either behind the eye or under the surface of the eye.

What happens during trabeculectomy

This technique is used to treat open-angle glaucoma. A trap-door flap is created in the sclera to help fluid drain. A peripheral iridectomy is performed at the same time.

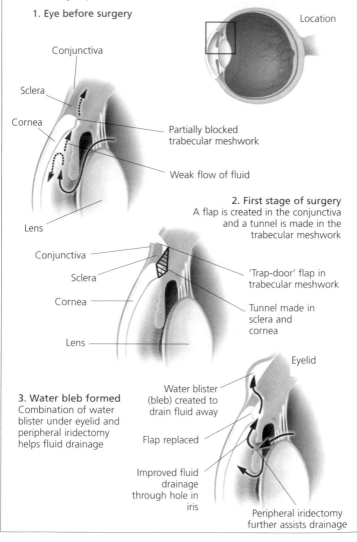

1. Eye before surgery

Location

Conjunctiva

Sclera

Cornea

Partially blocked trabecular meshwork

Weak flow of fluid

Lens

2. First stage of surgery
A flap is created in the conjunctiva and a tunnel is made in the trabecular meshwork

Conjunctiva

Sclera

Cornea

'Trap-door' flap in trabecular meshwork

Tunnel made in sclera and cornea

Lens

Eyelid

3. Water bleb formed
Combination of water blister under eyelid and peripheral iridectomy helps fluid drainage

Water blister (bleb) created to drain fluid away

Flap replaced

Improved fluid drainage through hole in iris

Peripheral iridectomy further assists drainage

This procedure needs to be carried out in an operating theatre but can be done as a day case. It takes about 10 minutes and may make your eye ache for a few hours afterwards. Anti-inflammatory and antibiotic drops and pain relief are administered after the procedure.

Diode laser treatment works by applying energy to the ciliary body, thereby damaging the process by which the aqueous fluid is produced and in turn reducing the intraocular pressure. Although it is extremely effective in reducing pressure, the ciliary body often repairs itself and the pressure rises once again, requiring repeat diode laser treatment. Sometimes four or five treatments may be required.

Combined trabeculectomy with cataract surgery

If you have glaucoma that is not satisfactorily controlled with drops and you have cataracts, your eye surgeon may recommend that you have an operation that combines cataract surgery with trabeculectomy. This is a well-recognised procedure that provides the benefit of the trabeculectomy and the cataract surgery in one operation. The operation takes slightly longer than trabeculectomy alone and may take up to an hour. This can be carried out under a local or a general anaesthetic (see page 59).

Benefits and risk of surgery for glaucoma

Any form of surgery carries a small risk and should be carried out only after the benefits of the surgery have been carefully weighed against the potential risks. You should discuss with your eye specialist the indications for surgical treatment, its benefits and risks.

Diode laser treatment

The laser is directed at the ciliary body, damaging the process by which the aqueous fluid is produced, so reducing the amount of fluid produced and therefore the pressure in the eye.

Location

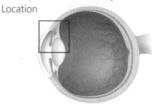

1. Before surgery
Normal quantities of aqueous fluid produced but it cannot drain

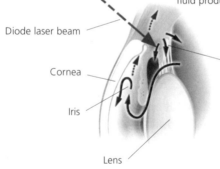

Weak flow of fluid through meshwork

Partially blocked trabecular meshwork

2. Damage to ciliary body
The laser beam is directed at the ciliary body to reduce amount of fluid produced

Diode laser beam

Ciliary body producing aqueous fluid

Cornea

Iris

Lens

Fluid drains easily

Production of aqueous fluid is reduced

3. After treatment
As the ciliary body produces less fluid, it can drain easily through the trabecular meshwork

Questions to ask your consultant

- What benefits should the surgery provide?
- What are the risks if surgery isn't performed?
- How many of these procedures have you carried out? With what results?
- What are the possible risks and complications?
- How long will I need to stay in hospital?
- How long will it take my eye to heal?
- Will my vision change?
- Are there any activities that I should avoid afterwards?
- Will I need ongoing medication?
- Will I need new glasses after the operation?

Pros and cons of trabeculectomy

Trabeculectomy successfully controls the intraocular pressure in the great majority of cases. The treatment is often so successful that eyedrops can be stopped.

The side effects of trabeculectomy, on the other hand, can include bleeding within the eye at the time of surgery (known as hyphaema); this usually clears readily after a few days, although it can cause blurred vision in the meantime.

Another potential side effect happens when the drainage bleb is too effective and drains the fluid out of the eye too quickly, making the eye softer than it should be. Once again this is usually self-limiting and the problem resolves as the operation heals.

Surgery for open-angle glaucoma can predispose to the development of a cataract in the eye, although this can usually be treated with cataract surgery (see page 44).

Over the first few years there is an increasing risk that the trabeculectomy bleb can heal over and stop functioning. Premature healing of the bleb is particularly prevalent in patients of African origin or in people below the age of 40.

Under these circumstances the surgeon may opt to use special drops (an antimetabolite) during surgery that reduce the risk of premature healing, but this can sometimes lead to over-draining of the bleb. If the bleb heals over and stops functioning, it can be opened up again by the surgeon using a simple procedure under local anaesthetic ('needling' – see page 96). Infection of the eye (endophthalmitis) is a rare complication of trabeculectomy.

Assessment before the operation

This is similar to that required for cataract surgery (see page 44), apart from the fact that the surgeon does not need to measure the length of your eye. Your eyes will be examined before the operation to check that there are no potential sources of infection such as conjunctivitis and blepharitis (infection of the lids), which would need to be treated with antibiotics before surgery would be considered.

Equally any source of infection elsewhere in the body such as a urinary infection or leg ulcer would also need to be treated. It is important to let your eye surgeon know if you believe that you have any of these potential sources of infection because of the risk of contamination during surgery.

The anaesthetic

For a trabeculectomy or combined trabeculectomy and cataract surgery, a local or general anaesthetic is required and is identical to the anaesthetic used in cataract surgery (see page 59).

Postoperative recovery and treatment

Most people have a pad put on the eye for a few hours after the operation and when this is removed vision may initially be quite blurred. Your sight should gradually improve over the first postoperative week but you may need new glasses, so you should go to your optometrist about one month after the surgery or as advised by your eye surgeon.

Medication after surgery

Your eye surgeon will probably want to see you the day after the operation and then again approximately one week and four weeks after the operation. During this period your eye will be treated with antibiotic and steroid or other anti-inflammatory drops, but you will not need to continue with the glaucoma drops for the eye that has been operated upon. Your glaucoma drops will, however, be necessary for the other eye if it has not had surgery, and you need to seek the advice of the eye surgeon about this point.

Your eye may ache a little after the operation but this is usually satisfactorily controlled with a mild oral pain relief in combination with the prescribed drops. Recovery of the eye is otherwise similar to that after cataract surgery (see page 61) and most people can return to work after approximately two weeks.

Once again heavy lifting and straining need to be avoided for the first six weeks after surgery as this can cause a rise in pressure in the eye that could potentially damage the wound.

If all is well at the time of your one-month postoperative appointment, your surgeon will probably return to the previous pattern of monitoring the glaucoma as an outpatient two to three times a year.

Further treatment

As mentioned previously, over the years the bleb formed during trabeculectomy can gradually heal over. If this occurs it can be repeated or sometimes your surgeon will carry out a simple 'needling' procedure. This involves inserting a needle into the bleb and breaking down the scar tissue to allow the bleb to function satisfactorily once again. This is carried out under a local anaesthetic and can be done as an outpatient procedure or sometimes as a day case in the operating theatre. This procedure is simple and more straightforward than the original trabeculectomy operation.

KEY POINTS

■ Surgery for glaucoma (trabeculectomy) is usually straightforward and has good results

■ Serious complications are rare

■ Laser treatment is also available but is usually reserved for those cases where drainage surgery (trabeculectomy) has already been tried

■ After successful glaucoma surgery, the glaucoma treatment drops can usually be discontinued for the operated eye, but will need to be continued in the other eye if this has not had surgery

■ After surgery the glaucoma still needs to be monitored with outpatient appointments two to three times a year

Macular degeneration

What is macular degeneration?

This is an eye condition that affects the central (reading) part of sight. It is the most common cause of poor eyesight in people aged over 60. It never leads to complete sight loss, because it is only the central vision that is affected. However, in many cases, it is difficult or impossible to treat.

It is caused by disease changes at the most highly developed part of the retina (the macula), which is made up of millions of light-sensitive cone and rod cells. The macula is situated at the centre of your retina at the point where most of the light rays coming into the eye are focused. It is responsible for your central vision, for detailed visual activities, such as reading and writing, and your ability to appreciate colour.

In macular degeneration the highly specialised photoreceptor cells in the macula stop functioning, either partially or completely. Macular degeneration usually affects both eyes, although it tends to be asymmetrical – meaning that it affects one eye more than the other.

Types of macular degeneration

Age-related macular degeneration is by far the most common form of the disease and it affects about 500,000 people in the UK. It mostly affects people aged over 60 and is more common with increasing age. Other conditions such as macular dystrophies (see later) are much rarer and tend to affect younger people.

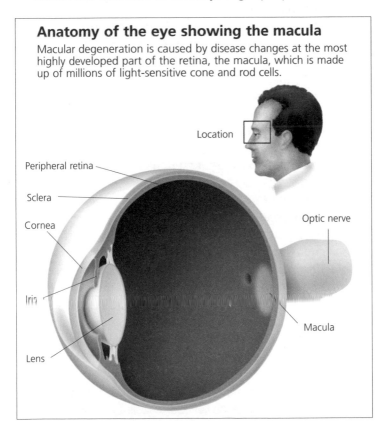

Anatomy of the eye showing the macula

Macular degeneration is caused by disease changes at the most highly developed part of the retina, the macula, which is made up of millions of light-sensitive cone and rod cells.

Location

Peripheral retina

Sclera

Cornea

Optic nerve

Iris

Macula

Lens

Age-related macular degeneration

This can be loosely divided into two main types: the 'dry form' and the 'wet form'. The dry form, which cannot be treated, develops slowly. It is caused by a gradual failure of the delicate cells that control the central vision at the macula. It is more common than the wet form of the disease and is not associated with water logging or bleeding at the macula – hence the description of the condition as 'dry'.

Dry-form degeneration

In dry-form age-related macular degeneration, important supporting cells of the retina (retinal pigment epithelial or RPE cells) start to malfunction and die and can lead to patches of atrophy (dead areas, like a worn carpet) interspersed by pigment clumping with a characteristic appearance. As the retinal pigment epithelial cells die off there is an associated loss of the retinal photoreceptor cells (the rods and cones), thus resulting in a reduction in central macular vision.

Wet-form degeneration

The wet variety (seen in less than 20 per cent of cases) can have a much more rapid effect on your eyesight, sometimes causing a severe loss of central vision within a matter of days. It is caused by the growth of abnormal blood vessels through age-related defects in the deepest layer of the retina (usually in the macular region). These abnormal vessels form a membrane called a 'choroidal neovascular membrane'. These vessels can leak, causing water logging of the macula, which affects your central vision. In addition, these vessels are fragile and can bleed, causing scarring.

The wet variety of macular degeneration is also known as a 'disciform maculopathy' or a 'subretinal neovascular membrane'. It can occasionally be treated with laser therapy which ablates, or destroys, the blood vessels closing them off (see page 108).

What causes age-related macular degeneration?
The precise cause is unknown. It is thought to be related to the genetic 'clock' of the specialist macular cells, which start functioning abnormally and eventually die. The dry form usually occurs before the wet variety and both frequently coexist.

Age-related changes at the macula are often seen in eyes of people over the age of 60, commonly in people with normal vision. These changes do not always lead to the degenerative changes that reduce sight. The most common age-related finding at the macula are yellowish-white spots in the retina called 'drusen'. These represent an accumulation of the by-products of the metabolism of the retina in the deepest layer of the retina (Bruch's membrane) and are associated with a failure of retinal pigment epithelial cells.

Drusen are divided into two varieties according to their appearance: 'soft drusen', which are round and less distinct than the other variety, and 'hard drusen', which have a glinting appearance. Drusen alone do not affect visual function, but may forewarn of the development of dry or wet macular degeneration as described above. This is more likely with soft rather than hard drusen. The detailed diagnosis of this condition is specialised and requires an examination by a hospital eye specialist.

Risk factors

Age-related macular degeneration may also be more common in some families, although a precise pattern of inheritance has not been determined and most cases have no family history. Smoking has been identified as a predisposing factor and more than doubles the risk of advanced age-related macular degeneration. If you have a family history of macular degeneration you should not smoke. There is also some evidence that high cholesterol levels in the blood contribute to the development of macular degeneration.

Macular dystrophies

These develop when the specialist cells in the macula stop working normally. They are much rarer than age-related macular degeneration and often affect people at a younger age. Many macular dystrophies are inherited, or congenital, and in these forms it is believed that the malfunction is the result of defects in the genetic make-up of the cells.

Other causes of macular disease

Injury or trauma (usually involving a direct blow to the eye) can damage the macula and lead to macular degenerative changes at the time or later in life.

Some medications have been linked to macular damage, but usually only in very high doses. These include antidepressants (such as chlorpromazine), drugs used in the prevention and treatment of malaria (such as chloroquine), tamoxifen (used in the treatment of some breast cancers) and some medicines used to treat rheumatoid arthritis (hydroxychloroquine and chloroquine). If you are worried about whether your medicines can cause or worsen macular degeneration, you should read the information leaflet provided with them. If this leaflet suggests macular degeneration and/or damage to the macula as a potential side effect, you should seek advice from your GP or hospital eye specialist.

Short-sightedness (myopia) can predispose a person to the development of macular degeneration, which usually comes on later in life. However, in this group it can occur at a younger age than 'age-related' macular degeneration. The precise mechanism for this is not fully understood.

Age-related macular degeneration
Who is affected?

As described, this becomes increasingly common as people age. However, many people have signs of ageing at the macula but retain good sight. Both men and women are affected equally and there do not appear to be any particular differences between different races or geographical origins. Age-related macular degeneration can coexist with cataracts and/or glaucoma, but these conditions do not predispose to the development of macular disease.

Possible symptoms

In the early stages, you may notice that images are blurred or distorted (for example, straight lines may look kinked) and that there is a change in the size of the image, with objects looking smaller or larger than with the other eye. You may also find that reading becomes difficult and that you miss out letters or words.

If only one eye is affected, you may not notice the early symptoms. However, later on, your vision may be further affected so that there appears to be a blank spot or dark patch in the centre of your visual field, faces are difficult to recognise and reading is even more difficult. Driving may not be possible. Some people with macular degeneration notice a dark patch in the centre of their vision when they wake in the morning, but find that this patch gradually fades over about half an hour.

Your appreciation of colour may be affected, although this may not be noticeable. Your eyes may be sensitive to bright light and, if the condition is advanced, flashes of light or unusual images may be seen. Your detailed central vision may be particularly poor in low lighting. Although your central vision may eventually be lost, people with macular degeneration alone never lose their eyesight completely because the peripheral (side) vision is always retained. This means that almost everyone with macular degeneration will have enough sight to get about without help and can maintain their independence.

If you notice a sudden onset of any of the above symptoms, particularly distortion in your central vision, you should seek urgent advice from your optometrist and/or your doctor, who will refer you to an ophthalmologist or the eye accident and emergency department as necessary. If symptoms develop suddenly it can indicate the beginnings of the wet form of macular degeneration, which can, occasionally, be treated with a laser.

Diagnosis

Macular degenerative changes may first be noticed by your optometrist and/or your GP during a routine eye examination and can occur before any of the associated symptoms arise. If these changes are significant and/or you are experiencing symptoms, you will usually be referred to an ophthalmologist to confirm the diagnosis.

This usually involves a comprehensive examination of the eye, including the dilation (widening) of the pupils with drops to give the ophthalmologist a better view of your retina. These drops will blur your vision so you will not be able to drive for six to eight hours afterwards and should arrange for someone to take you home.

Examination with an angiogram

If the wet form of macular degeneration is suspected, a fundus fluorescein angiogram (FFA) may be performed. A fluorescent dye (fluorescein) is injected into a vein in your arm and a series of colour photographs of the retina taken as the dye passes through the blood vessels in the back of the eye. These photographs provide an accurate map of the changes occurring at the macula, and help your ophthalmologist decide whether you have the 'dry' or 'wet' form of the disease, and whether laser treatment is possible.

The angiogram usually takes less than 10 minutes to perform. It is not painful, but may make you feel light-headed or a little nauseous, and the light from the camera can be quite dazzling for a few minutes afterwards. The dye used for the injection causes a transient yellow discolouration of the skin, and turns your urine yellow for 24 hours.

Treatment
How you can help yourself
There is usually no medical treatment for the dry form

Fundus fluorescein angiogram

Also called an FFA, this can be used to study the blood vessels at the back of the eye. A fluorescent dye is injected into the arm, and a series of photographs taken as the dye flows through the blood vessels in the back of the eye.

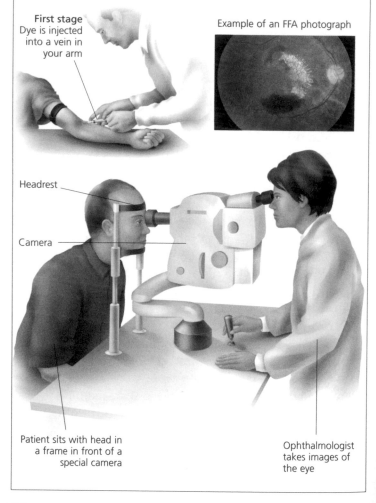

First stage
Dye is injected into a vein in your arm

Example of an FFA photograph

Headrest

Camera

Patient sits with head in a frame in front of a special camera

Ophthalmologist takes images of the eye

of macular degeneration. However, if you are diagnosed with macular degeneration you should give up smoking. You should also have your cholesterol levels checked and, if high, take steps to lower them with diet or you may be given medication (a statin) by your doctor. It has been suggested that in advanced disease dietary supplements of antioxidant vitamins A, C and E and zinc may be helpful.

More recently there has been some weak evidence to support treatment with dietary carotenoids called lutein and zeaxanthin, which are also antioxidants. It is known that lutein is present in large quantities in the normal macular tissue, and is readily available in the diet, particularly in red and green peppers, sweetcorn, spinach and eggs.

There are a number of commercially available tablets containing vitamins A, C and E, and zinc, lutein and zeaxanthin. A healthy diet rich in green vegetables should be sufficient without the use of supplements. Check with your doctor before taking supplements.

It is worth noting that only one scientific study (the Age-Related Eye Disease Study or AREDS) found evidence to support the use of high doses of zinc, and the antioxidant vitamins A, C and E were shown to be helpful wherever marked age-related degenerative changes were found in one eye. Vitamin A supplements should not be taken by people who smoke, because there is evidence that this could increase the risk of lung cancer.

Anti-vascular endothelial growth factor treatment (anti-VEGF)

In September 2008 the National Institute for Health and Clinical Excellence (NICE) approved the use of ranibizumab (Lucentis) for treatment of the wet variety

of age-related macular degeneration. This consists of
an injection into the eye of the substance, which shrinks
the abnormal blood vessels in the retina that are causing
the wet macular degeneration. It is suitable only for
people whose vision is not too severely affected (Snellen
visual acuity of 6/96 or better), where the lesion is not
too large and where there has not been significant
bleeding in the macular region.

The outcome of treatment is encouraging and will
improve vision to an extent in some patients. It does not
usually restore vision completely. The treatment often has
to be repeated and on average 5.2 treatments are
needed in the first year. If you have wet macular
degeneration, please ask your eye specialist whether your
eye would be amenable to this form of treatment.

Argon-laser therapy

For the wet form of macular degeneration, argon
(thermal) laser treatment can occasionally delay the
progression of the disease but is appropriate only in
about 10 per cent of cases.

If the subretinal membrane of blood vessels (choroidal
neovascular membrane) impinges on, or is very near to,
the very central part of the macula (the fovea), treatment
with argon laser to the membrane will usually destroy
the central vision and is therefore of no benefit.

If the membrane is situated away from the fovea,
argon laser treatment can be used to destroy and close
down the blood vessels in the offending membrane.
In these cases, the treatment is successful in about half
the patients, but unfortunately there is a 50 per cent
chance of recurrence within 3 years.

Laser treatment tends to lead to dying off (atrophy)
of the overlying retina in the region of the treatment,

and this may be noticed by the patient as a blank patch in his or her sight.

What happens during laser treatment

Laser treatment is carried out as an outpatient procedure. The pupil of the affected eye is dilated with drops. Local anaesthetic drops are then applied and a contact lens placed on the eye. As the local anaesthetic numbs the eye, you will not feel the contact lens and it keeps your eye open so you do not need to be concerned about blinking. The laser treatment is then applied while you sit in front of a slit-lamp biomicroscope (similar to that used to examine your eye).

The flashes of laser light are very bright and can lead to the eye being dazzled for half an hour or so after the procedure. Laser treatment of this kind is not painful. It is probably helpful to ask a friend or relative to accompany you to the hospital for laser treatment and you cannot drive until the effects of the dilating drops have worn off (six to eight hours), and then only if your sight is good enough. People who have the wet form of macular degeneration should discuss the possibility of treatment with their ophthalmologist.

Optical aids

Various aids are available for people with poor vision caused by macular degeneration and these are described in the next chapter (see page 119).

Monitoring macular degeneration

The dry form of macular degeneration usually progresses gradually and the eyesight is never lost completely as peripheral vision is retained. It is possible to monitor the condition by assessing changes in the symptoms, especially your close-up, or reading, vision. More formal monitoring of distance and reading sight can be done by your optometrist and/or ophthalmologist who can also chart changes in your retina. However, regular monitoring by the hospital specialists is not normally required.

A special chart is available from the eye consultant to help you monitor your eyesight (an Amsler chart). An example is shown opposite together with instructions for its use. The chart is particularly helpful in recognising the onset of distortion in the central vision. To use it, you need to wear reading glasses and test each eye separately (with your other eye covered with the palm of your hand).

The Amsler chart consists of a black central spot surrounded by a grid of horizontal and vertical black lines. Concentrate on the central black spot and assess whether any of the grid lines are distorted or any part of the image on the chart is missing.

Getting help

If you believe that you have macular degeneration or you have a family history of the disease, you should first visit your optometrist for a check-up, explaining your concerns and symptoms. If he or she believes that you have significant macular disease (or your symptoms persist), you should consult your doctor (your optometrist can refer you to your doctor) who can arrange an appointment with an ophthalmologist.

Sometimes, patients with wet macular degeneration in one eye are advised to phone their eye hospital accident and emergency department as soon as possible if they suddenly develop symptoms in the other eye. You should discuss this with your ophthalmologist.

Monitoring your eyesight

An Amsler chart can help you monitor your eyesight.

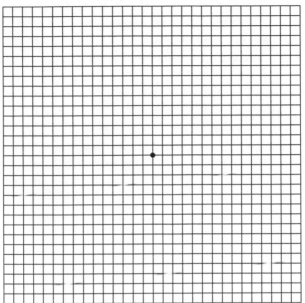

How to use the Amsler chart

1. Place this page at eye level and where light is consistent and without glare.
2. Put on your reading glasses and cover one eye.
3. Fix your gaze on the central black dot.
4. Keeping your gaze fixed, try to see if any lines are distorted or missing.
5. Mark the defect on the chart.
6. Test each eye separately.
7. If the distortion is new or has worsened, arrange to see your ophthalmologist urgently.
8. Always keep the Amsler chart the *same distance* from your eyes each time that you test.

Driving and macular degeneration

If your sight is affected by macular degeneration, driving may become more difficult, particularly at night, or in conditions of poor light. There are strict regulations laid down by law and administered by the Driver and Vehicle Licensing Agency (DVLA). Your sight does not need to have deteriorated very greatly to fail to achieve the legal visual requirements for driving. If you have doubts, you should visit your optometrist for a check-up and advice.

Many people with mild macular degeneration are able to drive normally, although some choose not to drive at night or when the lighting conditions are poor.

If you are advised that your sight does not meet the legal requirements for driving, you should inform the DVLA at Swansea (see page 126). You should also be aware that your car insurance is not valid if your vision falls below the legal standard.

Recent advances in treatment

Over the past few years, there has been a lot of interest and research in the treatment of age-related macular degeneration. Although there has been no significant progress in preventing the onset of the disease, there are a number of medical trials in progress concentrating on the treatment of the wet form of the disease. These potential new treatments include photodynamic therapy, anti-vascular endothelial growth factor treatment and radiotherapy.

Photodynamic therapy (PDT)

This is used to treat the wet form (exudative or neovascular disease) of macular degeneration and is appropriate only for certain cases (your ophthalmologist can advise you). It has no place in established damage from the wet-form macular degeneration or in the dry variety.

The treatment uses a cold laser beam (low energy), which does not damage normal retinal tissue. This contrasts with the high-energy, thermal, argon-laser therapy conventionally used only to treat disciform maculopathy that is situated well away from the very centre of the macula (the fovea).

Before treatment with the cold laser, a light-sensitive substance (photosensitive) is injected into a vein in your arm. This substance is derived from a group of naturally occurring compounds called 'porphyrins'. It concentrates in the abnormal blood vessels at the macula by attaching to the vessel walls, and allows energy from the laser to be targeted at the abnormal vascular membrane, thereby destroying it.

Although the vascular membrane regresses after the laser treatment, there is evidence that it tends to regrow within the first six months and to require further treatment. Repeated treatment can cause retinal thinning and loss of the specialist cells in the macula, mimicking the dry form of macular degeneration.

Long-term effects

It should be emphasised that photodynamic therapy cannot restore sight to a macula with established retinal damage. Treatment with photodynamic therapy is currently being evaluated in clinical trials on both sides of the Atlantic and much more work is required before definitive advice can be given about its effectiveness. Photodynamic therapy is now available within the NHS, but only for certain types of 'wet' macular degeneration. Your ophthalmologist will be able to advise you.

Anti-vascular endothelial growth factor treatment

Recent scientific studies into anti-vascular endothelial growth factors (anti-VEGFs) used to treat 'wet' macular degeneration have shown evidence that they may help to prevent deterioration in vision and even lead to some improvement in certain cases.

Treatment is designed to slow down the growth of the new vessels that form beneath the macula in wet-form age-related macular degeneration (choroidal neovascular membrane). At the moment it is not licensed for use in the UK. Treatment involves injections into the eye (into the 'vitreous humour' – see page 14). The injections may need to be carried out every six weeks.

Various side effects and complications have been reported including serious, albeit rare, problems such as infection inside the eye (endophthalmitis), retinal detachment or trauma-induced cataract. Ask your specialist hospital eye consultant if you wish to know more about this new treatment development.

Radiotherapy

Low-dose radiotherapy to the subretinal neovascular membrane has also been the subject of extensive research in recent years. However, although initial results were encouraging, it appears that the treatment damages the overlying retina as well as the affected membrane. Further evaluation is required before this form of treatment can be recommended.

Other treatments

Retinal translocation has excited considerable press interest, but is in the early stages of development. It involves moving the retinal tissue away from the underlying membrane before treating the membrane with a laser, therefore avoiding damage from the laser to the overlying retina.

It is appropriate only for a very small number of patients with the wet form of macular degeneration. Retinal translocation can cause double vision. Once again, this is not available as a routine NHS treatment and its efficacy is still being evaluated.

There is also some experimental work being carried out in animals involving the transplantation of parts of the retina, but the work is at a very early stage. In the distant future, gene therapy may be possible for people with a family history of the disease but, as a specific gene for age-related macular degeneration has yet to be identified, this form of potential therapy remains purely theoretical.

Long-term outlook for macular degeneration

It cannot be overemphasised that people with macular degeneration alone will never go blind. If people with this condition are registered as partially sighted or blind, it simply means that their central vision has deteriorated to a very low level.

Cataracts can often be present with macular degeneration and if these develop it may well be worth having cataract surgery in order to improve your vision. For more details, see 'Cataracts', page 34, and 'Cataract surgery', page 44. Your ophthalmologist can advise you.

KEY POINTS

- The most common form of macular degeneration is age related and affects people over the age of 60

- There are two main forms of age-related macular degeneration: 'wet' and 'dry'

- People with macular degeneration alone never lose their sight completely and will always retain their peripheral (navigational) vision

- There is no treatment for most forms of macular degeneration, but low vision aids (see page 119) can help the sight

- People with macular degeneration should not smoke

Registration as blind or partially sighted

Extra help is available

If you have very poor central vision and/or significant loss of visual field in both eyes, you can be registered as partially sighted or blind. This will enable you to obtain additional help and support from your local Social Services.

Registration can be arranged only by a hospital consultant ophthalmologist who, after examining your eyes, will complete the necessary paper work and forward it to the Department for the Visually Impaired at your local Social Services. The Social Services Officer will then get in touch with you and usually arrange a home visit to discuss placing you on the appropriate register. He or she will be able to tell you what is available in your area, for example, help at home, improved lighting and various home gadgets for people with poor sight.

As well as the benefits outlined in the box on pages 120–1, you may be entitled to financial help in the form of:

- Attendance Allowance (if you are over 65 years of age)
- Disability Living Allowance (if you are under 65)
- Carer's Allowance
- Incapacity Benefit
- Pension Credit
- Income Support
- Council Tax disability reduction
- Tax Credits: Working Tax Credit and Child Tax Credit.

This information is available on the RNIB's website: www.rnib.org.uk. For further information, contact your local Social Security Department, Citizens Advice Bureau (CAB), Welfare Rights Officer or Specialist Social Workers at Social Services. Also look at the RNIB's leaflet on free prescriptions and the Wales Council for the Blind's leaflet on disability. For contact details, please see Useful addresses, pages 130–2.

Aids for those with poor vision

There are also many practical aids that can be of help. These include talking watches, talking clocks, large dial telephones and timepieces. Advice as to where these can be found in your locality can be obtained from the specialist social workers at Social Services. Guide dogs can be immensely helpful and advice regarding the appropriateness and eligibility for a guide dog can be obtained from the Royal National Institute of Blind People (RNIB) – see page 131.

Glasses/Spectacles

If you have macular degeneration, you should ensure that your glasses are checked annually by your optometrist. This will ensure that you are getting the most out of your vision.

Low vision aids

These consist of very strong glasses (magnifying spectacles) and telescopes that enlarge the image to allow it to fall on the part of the retina not affected by the macular degenerative process. If a very large area of your retina is affected, these low vision aids are usually not helpful. The hospital eye specialist can refer those who would benefit from a trial of these aids to a specialist optometrist either in the community or in the hospital. Low vision aids are available free through the NHS although private assessments are also possible.

Closed circuit television systems (CCTV) may be of help in some circumstances. These consist of a video camera that will photograph a piece of text, magnify it and project it on to a screen. These systems are expensive and can cost up to £2,000; they are seldom available on the NHS. Once again advice about their availability can be obtained during a low vision aid assessment. The information may also be available through the local branch of the RNIB.

Books and newspapers

Large print books are available from all libraries and through most good book shops. Talking newspapers and talking books are also obtainable – more details are given in Useful addresses, pages 130 and 132.

Benefits of registering as blind or partially sighted

Benefit	Registered blind	Registered partially sighted
● Special blind person's personal income tax allowance	✔	✘
● Additional income support benefit (Attendance Allowance and Disability Living Allowance) *Apply to your local Benefit Agency or ring the Enquiry line on 0800 882 200*	✔	✘
● Exemption from 'Non-dependants' deductions from Income Support	✔	✘
● Additional Housing Benefit *Proof of Registration will be required when applying to the local housing department.*	✔	✔
● Exemption from 'Non-dependants' deductions	✔	**Possible**
● TV licence at reduced cost *Registered severely sight-impaired (blind) people are entitled to a 50 per cent annual reduction. A certificate will be issued by your local Social Services Department for you to take to the post office when you renew your licence. Ring TV licence helpline 0870 576 3763.*	✔	✘
● Postage concessions *Applies to certain articles including Braille material and spoken recordings, such as Talking Books and Talking Newspapers, but not personal tapes or typed letters. Details are available from the Royal National Institute of Blind People.*	✔	✔

Benefits of registering as blind or partially sighted (contd)

Benefit	Registered blind	Registered partially sighted
• Assistance with telephone costs	✔	✔

Financial assistance by the Social Services Department towards the cost of installing a telephone may be given in cases that meet the criteria for the Chronically Sick and Disabled Persons Act 1970. Applications are subject to an assessment of need.

• Telephones for the Blind Fund	✔	✘

This is a national charity that may give financial assistance in some cases. Apply to your local Social Services Department, where your application will be assessed against the criteria laid down by the Telephones for the Blind Fund (www.tftb.org.uk).

• Free bus passes	✔	✘

These are available to any person over the age of 16 years who is registered blind. Apply to your local Social Services Department.

• Disabled Person's Car Badges	✔	✔

If you are registered blind you may apply for a Disabled Person's Car Badge under the Blue Badge scheme. Application forms are available from your local Social Services Department. People who are partially sighted may be eligible if they have an additional disability.

• Disabled Person's Railcard	✔	✔

One-third off price of certain rail tickets. Application forms are available from your local post office, and National Rail Enquiries on 0845 748 4950.

• Free eye test	✔	✔

National Health Service (NHS) Eye Examination Fee.

Check RNIB's website www.rnib.org.uk for further details.

Lighting

Good bright lighting is essential to get the best out of your sight. An anglepoise or standard lamp with a strong bulb is helpful for reading, sewing and close work. Halogen bulbs create a good light without the heat that accompanies conventional light bulbs. Good daylight is helpful, so many people read in front of a sunny window.

KEY POINTS

- If you have very poor central vision, you may be entitled to register as partially sighted or blind

- Visual aids, audio books and magazines are available for people with poor vision

- Good lighting can help people with poor vision to read and do close work more easily

Useful addresses

Where can I find out more?
We have included the following organisations because, on preliminary investigation, they may be of use to the reader. However, we do not have first-hand experience of each organisation and so cannot guarantee the organisation's integrity. The reader must therefore exercise his or her own discretion and judgement when making further enquiries.

Association of Blind and Partially Sighted Teachers and Students
BM Box 6727
London WC1N 3XX
Tel: 01484 690521
Website: www.abapstas.org.uk

Originally supporting visually impaired students, teachers and lecturers, now a national self-help organisation with main focus on education and employment. Organises days on study skills, teaching techniques and confidence building.

Benefits Enquiry Line
Tel: 0800 882200
Minicom: 0800 243355
Website: www.dwp.gov.uk
N. Ireland: 0800 220674

Government agency giving information and advice on sickness and disability benefits for people with disabilities and their carers.

Blood Pressure Association
60 Cranmer Terrace
London SW17 0QS
Tel: 020 8772 4994
Website: www.bpassoc.org.uk

For the best internet advice. Regularly issues press statements when any new information becomes available and has advice leaflets on all aspects of hypertension (for example, pregnancy, renal disease, heart disease). Raises public awareness about, and offers information and support to, people affected by high blood pressure and health-care professionals. Has a wide selection of literature and membership scheme. Please send large A4 SAE and two first-class stamps for information.

Calibre Cassette Library
New Road, Weston Turville
Aylesbury, Bucks HP22 5XQ
Tel: 01296 432339
Website: www.calibre.org.uk

Library of 7,000 titles of unabridged books available on standard cassettes. Proof of disability allows borrowing for members in return for voluntary donations.

Carers UK
20 Great Dover Street
London SE1 4LX
Tel: 020 7378 4999
Helpline: 0808 808 7777 (Wed, Thurs 10am–12 noon, 2–4pm)
Website: www.carersuk.org

Encourages carers to recognise their own needs. Offers information, advice and support to all people who are unpaid carers looking after others with medical or other problems. Branches organise activities to help carers, social events and helplines.

Citizens Advice Bureaux
Myddelton House, 115–123 Pentonville Road
London N1 9LZ
Tel: 020 7833 2181 (admin only)
Website: www.adviceguide.org.uk

HQ of national charity offering a wide variety of practical, financial and legal advice. Network of local charities throughout the UK listed in phone books and in *Yellow Pages* under 'C'.

Clinical Knowledge Summaries
Sowerby Centre for Health Informatics at Newcastle (SCHIN Ltd), Bede House, All Saints Business Centre
Newcastle upon Tyne NE1 2ES

Tel: 0191 243 6100
Website: www.cks.library.nhs.uk

A website mainly for GPs giving information for patients listed by disease plus named self-help organisations.

Disabled Living Foundation
380–384 Harrow Road
London W9 2HU
Tel: 020 7289 6111
Helpline: 0845 130 9177
Textphone: 020 7432 8009
Website: www.dlf.org.uk

Provides information to disabled and elderly people on all kinds of equipment in order to promote their independence and quality of life.

Driver and Vehicle Licensing Agency (DVLA)
Driver Medical Section
Swansea SA6 7JL
Helpline: 0870 600 0301 (8am–5.30pm)
Website: www.dvla.gov.uk

Government office offering advice to drivers with medical conditions.

Great Ormond Street Hospital for Children NHS Trust
Great Ormond Street
London WC1N 3JH
Tel: 020 7405 9200
Website: www.gosh.nhs.uk

Information leaflets on childhood diseases, jointly compiled by the Institute of Child Health and Great Ormond Street Hospital for Children, are available via the former's website (see below).

Guide Dogs for the Blind Association
Burghfield Common
Reading RG7 3YG
Tel: 0118 983 5555
Website: www.guidedogs.org.uk

Provides guide dogs, mobility and other rehabilitation services to enable blind and partially sighted people to lead the fullest and most independent lives possible.

Institute of Child Health
30 Guilford Street
London WC1N 1EH
Tel: 020 7242 9789
Website: www.gosh.nhs.uk

See Great Ormond Street Hospital for Children NHS Trust.

LOOK, National Federation of Families with Visually Impaired Children
c/o Queen Alexandra College, 49 Court Oak Road
Harborne, Birmingham B17 9TG
Tel: 0121 428 5038
Website: www.look-uk.org

Offers information, help and support for parents who have visually impaired children; access to benefits, education and grants. Runs youth project for young people aged 9–18 years.

Macular Disease Society
PO Box 1870
Andover, Hants SP10 9AD
Tel: 01264 350551
Helpline: 0845 241 2041 (Mon–Fri, 9am–5pm)
Website: www.maculardisease.org

Provides information, a regular magazine available in large print or on audio-tape, and practical support for people with any of the eye conditions covered by the term 'macular disease'. Has local self-help branches and promotes research into macular disease.

National Institute for Health and Clinical Excellence (NICE)
MidCity Place, 71 High Holborn
London WC1V 6NA
Tel: 0845 003 7780
Website: www.nice.org.uk

Provides national guidance on the promotion of good health and the prevention and treatment of ill health. Patient information leaflets are available for each piece of guidance issued.

NHS Direct
Tel: 0845 4647 (24 hours, 365 days a year)
Website: www.nhsdirect.nhs.uk

Offers confidential health-care advice, information and referral service. A good first port of call for any health advice.

NHS Smoking Helplines
Freephone: 0800 169 0169

(7am–11pm, 365 days a year)
Website: www.gosmokefree.nhs.uk
Pregnancy smoking helpline: 0800 169 9169
(12 noon–9pm, 365 days a year)

Have advice, help and encouragement on giving up
smoking. Specialist advisers available to offer on-going
support to those who genuinely are trying to give up
smoking. Can refer to local branches.

Patients' Association
PO Box 935
Harrow, Middlesex HA1 3YJ
Helpline: 0845 608 4455
Tel: 020 8423 9111
Website: www.patients-association.com

Provides advice on patients' rights, leaflets and a
directory of self-help groups.

Quit (Smoking Quitlines)
211 Old Street
London EC1V 9NR
Helpline: 0800 002200 (9am–9pm, 365 days a year)
Tel: 020 7251 1551
Website: www.quit.org.uk
Scotland: 0800 848484
Wales: 0800 169 0169 (NHS)

Offers individual advice on giving up smoking in
English and Asian languages. Talks to schools on
smoking and pregnancy and can refer to local support
groups. Runs training courses for professionals.

RNIB Talking Books Service
PO Box 173
Peterborough PE2 6WS
Tel: 0173 337 5350
Helpline: 0845 762 6843 (Mon-Fri 8am–6pm, Sat 9am–4pm)
Customer services: 0845 702 3153
Minicom: 0845 758 5691
Website: www.rnib.org.uk/talkingbooks

For annual membership fee (£70 in 2006) offers loan of CD player and talking books.

Royal College of Ophthalmologists
17 Cornwall Terrace
London NW1 4QW
Tel: 020 7935 0702
Website: www.rcophth.ac.uk

Professional college for eye specialists which produces a number of leaflets about a variety of eye diseases.

Royal National Institute of Blind People (RNIB)
105 Judd Street
London WC1H 9NE
Tel: 020 7388 1266
Welfare Rights Service: 0845 766 9999
Helpline: 0303 123 9999 (Mon–Fri, 9am–5pm)
Website: www.rnib.org.uk

Campaigns on behalf of people with sight problems and funds research. Offers a range of information and advice on lifestyle changes and employment for people facing loss of sight. Give advice on benefits just to those with sight loss, their carers or dependants. Also offers support and training in Braille and computers. Has mail order catalogue of useful aids. Has branches in Wales, Scotland and Northern Ireland (see below).

Royal National Institute of Blind People, Cymru
Trident Court, East Moors Road
Cardiff CF24 5TD
Tel: 029 2045 0440
Helpline: 0303 123 9999 (Mon–Fri, 9am–5pm)
Website: www.rnib.org.uk

Royal National Institute of Blind People, N. Ireland
40 Linenhall Street
Belfast BT2 8BA
Tel: 028 9032 9373
Website: www.rnib.org.uk

Royal National Institute of Blind People, Scotland
Dunedin House, 25 Ravelston Terrace
Edinburgh EH4 3TP
Tel: 0131 311 8500
Website: www.rnib.org.uk

Sense
101 Pentonville Road
London N1 9LG
Tel: 0845 127 0060
Textphone: 0845 127 0062
Website: www.sense.org.uk

Offers information, advice and support to people who are deaf–blind and those suffering from rubella and associated disabilities. Can refer for assessment as appropriate. Has branches in various parts of the UK (see below).

Sense Scotland
43 Middlesex Street
Kinning Park
Glasgow G41 1EE
Tel: 0141 429 0294
Textphone: 0141 418 7170
Website: www.sensescotland.org.uk

Talking Newspaper Association UK (TNAUK)
National Recording Centre, Browning Road
Heathfield, E. Sussex TN21 8DB
Tel: 01435 866102
Website: www.tnauk.org.uk

Lists 200 national newspapers and magazines on audio-tape, computer disk, CD-ROM and email for loan to visually impaired, blind and physically disabled people. Subscription from £30 annually.

Wales Council for the Blind
3rd Floor, Shand House, 20 Newport Road
Cardiff CF24 0DB
Tel: 029 2047 3954
Website: www.wcb-ccd.org.uk

Charity umbrella body for visually impaired organisations and local authorities in Wales. Information on benefits and general welfare as well as training for professionals and technological advice for visually impaired people. Transcription service available.

The internet as a further source of information

After reading this book, you may feel that you would like further information on the subject. The internet is of course an excellent place to look and there are many websites with useful information about medical disorders, related charities and support groups.

For those who do not have a computer at home some bars and cafes offer facilities for accessing the internet. These are listed in the *Yellow Pages* under 'Internet Bars and Cafes' and 'Internet Providers'. Your local library offers a similar facility and has staff to help you find the information that you need.

It should always be remembered, however, that the internet is unregulated and anyone is free to set up a website and add information to it. Many websites offer impartial advice and information that has been compiled and checked by qualified medical professionals. Some, on the other hand, are run by commercial organisations with the purpose of promoting their own products. Others still are run by pressure groups, some of which will provide carefully assessed and accurate information whereas others may be suggesting medications or treatments that are not supported by the medical and scientific community.

Unless you know the address of the website you want to visit – for example, www.familydoctor.co.uk – you may find the following guidelines useful when searching the internet for information.

Search engines and other searchable sites

Google (www.google.co.uk) is the most popular search engine used in the UK, followed by Yahoo! (http://uk.yahoo.com) and MSN (www.msn.co.uk). Also popular are the search engines provided by Internet Service Providers such as Tiscali and other sites such as the BBC site (www.bbc.co.uk).

In addition to the search engines that index the whole web, there are also medical sites with search facilities, which act almost like mini-search engines, but cover only medical topics or even a particular area of medicine. Again, it is wise to look at who is responsible for compiling the information offered to ensure that it is impartial and medically accurate. The NHS Direct site (www.nhsdirect. nhs.uk) is an example of a searchable medical site.

Links to many British medical charities can be found at the Association of Medical Research Charities website (www.amrc.org.uk) and at Charity Choice (www.charitychoice.co.uk).

Search phrases

Be specific when entering a search phrase. Searching for information on 'cancer' will return results for many different types of cancer as well as on cancer in general. You may even find sites offering astrological information. More useful results will be returned by using search phrases such as 'lung cancer' and 'treatments for lung cancer'. Both Google and Yahoo! offer an advanced search option that includes the ability to search for the exact phrase, enclosing the search phrase in quotes, that is, 'treatments for lung cancer' will have the same effect. Limiting a search to an exact phrase reduces the number of results returned but it is best to refine a search to an exact match only if you are not getting useful results with a normal search. Adding 'UK' to your search term will bring up mainly British sites, so a good phrase might be 'lung cancer' UK (don't include UK within the quotes).

Always remember the internet is international and unregulated. It holds a wealth of valuable information but individual sites may be biased, out of date or just plain wrong. Family Doctor Publications accepts no responsibility for the content of links published in this series.

Index

accommodation (focusing)
    16, 17
  – artificial lenses 47, 54
acetazolamide 81, 82, 84
aching of eye
  – in angle-closure
    glaucoma 83
  – after cataract surgery 62,
    65
  – after glaucoma surgery
    95
  – as side effect of
    medication 80
adrenaline (epinephrine) eye-
    drops 81
African origins, risk of
    glaucoma 75
age-related cataracts 35
Age-Related Eye Disease
    Study (AREDS) 107
age-related macular
    degeneration 4, 100–1,
    116
  – causes 101
  – diagnosis 104–5
  – driving 112

  – getting help 110
  – glasses 119
  – long-term outlook 115
  – monitoring 109–10, 111
  – risk factors 102
  – symptoms 103–4
  – treatment 105, 107–9,
    112–15
  – who is affected 103
  – see also macular
    degeneration
ageing
  – association with
    glaucoma 75
  – effect on eyes 1, 23, 32
aids for those with poor
    vision 118–19, 122
allergies 56
  – to eyedrops 82
allowances 118, 120–1
alpha-2 agonists 82
Amsler charts 110, 111
anaesthetics
  – for cataract surgery
    58–60
  – for trabeculectomy 94–5

angiograms 105, 106
angle-closure glaucoma 71, 72, 74, 87
 – causes 83
 – diagnosis 84
 – symptoms 83–4
 – treatment 84–5
 – see also glaucoma
anisometropia 54
anterior chamber 16, 39
antidepressants, link to macular damage 102
anti-inflammatories, for angle-closure glaucoma 85
anti-malarials, link to macular damage 102
antioxidant vitamin supplements 107
anti-vascular endothelial growth factor treatment 107–8, 114
apraclonidine 82
aqueous humour 14, 16, 39
 – production and drainage 71–2, 74
argon-laser therapy, macular degeneration 108–9
artificial lenses 47
 – selection of lens 53–4
artificial tears 12
 – see also intraocular lens implantation
Association of Blind and Partially Sighted Teachers and Students 123
Association of Medical Research Charities 134
asthma 79, 80
astigmatism 31
 – after cataract surgery 49

atropine (belladonna) eyedrops 15
Attendance Allowance 120

babies
 – congenital cataracts 35
 – glaucoma 73
bathing after cataract surgery 64
belladonna eyedrops 15
benefits 118, 120–1
Benefits Enquiry Line 124
beta blockers 80
betaxolol 80
bifocal lenses 27
bimatoprost 79
biometry testing 52–3
blank spots in field of vision 104
bleb, trabeculectomy 88, 90
 – premature healing 94, 96
bleeding after cataract surgery 64
blindness, registration 117–18
Blood Pressure Association 124
blood tests
 – monitoring medication 81, 82
 – preoperative 55
Blue Badge scheme 121
blurring of vision
 – in age-related macular degeneration 102
 – in angle-closure glaucoma 83, 84
 – cataracts as cause 38, 40
 – as side effect of medication 80
books, large print 119
brain, interpretation of visual signals 20

bright light, sensitivity to 40
brimonidine 82
brinzolamide 81
Bruch's membrane 101
bus passes 121

Calibre Cassette Library 124–5
capsule of lens 39
carbachol 80
carbonic anhydrase inhibitors 81, 82
Carers UK 125
carteolol 80
cataract surgery 2–3, 44, 69
– anaesthetics 58–60
– benefits and risks 51–2
– combination with trabeculectomy 91
– day case or overnight stay 57–8
– extracapsular 47–9
– intracapsular 49–51
– new glasses 66–8
– the operation 60–1
– phacoemulsification 45–7
– possible complications 64–6
– postoperative recovery and treatment 61–4
– questions to ask your consultant 57
– small incision non-phacoemulsification surgery 47
– treatment of refractive errors 32
cataracts 1, 2, 9
– appearance 37
– assessment for surgery 52–6
– causes 34–6
– coexistence with macular degeneration 5, 115
– diagnosis 41
– driving 43
– requirement for treatment 42
– risk after glaucoma surgery 93
– safety of treatment 42
– as side effect of medication 81
– symptoms 38, 40–1
– types 36–8
– what they are 34
Charity Choice 134
chloroquine, link to macular damage 102
chlorpromazine 102
cholesterol levels, relationship to macular degeneration 102, 107
choroid 14
choroidal neovascular membrane 100
chronic obstructive pulmonary disease (COPD) 80
ciliary body 14, 16, 18, 39
– diode laser treatment 91, 92
ciliary muscles 16, 17
Citizens Advice Bureaux 125
Clinical Knowledge Summaries 125–6
closed-angle glaucoma see angle-closure glaucoma
closed circuit television systems (CCTV) 119
colour blindness 19

colour vision 19
– effect of cataracts 37, 40
– effect of macular
degeneration 104
cone photoreceptors 18, 19
congenital cataracts 35
conjunctiva 12, 14
consultant ophthalmologists
5–6
cornea 12–13, 14, 18
cortical cataracts 37
– symptoms 40
cupping of optic nerve 76

dark patches in field of vision
104
day-case cataract surgery 58
dazzling 40
diabetes 26
– as cause of cataracts 36,
38
dietary supplements 107
diode laser treatment 89,
91, 92
dipivefrine eyedrops 81
Disability Living Allowance
120
Disabled Living Foundation
126
disabled person's car badges
121
disciform maculopathy see
wet-form age-related
macular degeneration
dispensing opticians 7
distorted images 103
doctors 8
– consultant
ophthalmologists 5–6
dorzolamide 81
double vision
– after cataract surgery 62

– as symptom of cataracts
37, 40
drainage angle 16, 71, 74
drinking before surgery 59,
60
driving
– after cataract surgery 63
– and cataracts 43
– after dilation of pupils 41
– and glaucoma 85–6
– and macular
degeneration 112
drusen 101
dry eyes, as side effect of
medication 80
dry-form age-related macular
degeneration 100
– see also macular
degeneration
DVLA (Driver and Vehicle
Licensing Authority) 126
– informing them about
eye conditions 86, 112

eating before surgery 59, 60
electrocardiogram (ECG),
preoperative 55–6
endophthalmitis 65, 94
epinephrine (adrenaline)
eyedrops 81
examination of the eyes
– before cataract surgery
52–3
– in glaucoma 76–9
– see also eye tests
extracapsular cataract surgery
47–9
eye care 28–9
eyedrops
– after cataract surgery 62
– for angle-closure
glaucoma 84–5

eyedrops (contd)
 – for open-angle glaucoma
  79–82
eye movements 12, 13
eye shields, use after cataract
  surgery 64
eye tests 23–4
 – free 26, 121
 – health checks 26
 – refraction test 27
 – Snellen chart 25
 – visual acuity tests 24–6
eyelashes, effect of
  prostaglandin drops 80
eyelids, function 11
eyes
 – focusing 16, 17
 – how they work 10, 18, 20
 – protection 10–11
 – structure 14

family history of eye disease
 – glaucoma 73, 75
 – macular degeneration
  102
fibres of lens 39
fields of vision 20–1
'floaters' 19
focusing (accommodation)
  16, 17
 – artificial lenses 47, 54
fovea 14, 18
free eye tests 26, 121
front (anterior) chamber 16,
  39
fundus fluorescein angiogram
  (FFA) 105, 106

general anaesthetics 59–60
general practice, eye care 28
generic names 79
German measles (rubella) 35

ghosting, as symptom of
  cataracts 37, 40
glasses
 – after cataract surgery 63,
  66–8
 – for long-sightedness 29,
  30
 – for those with macular
  degeneration 119
 – for short-sightedness 29,
  30, 31
 – types of lens 27–8
glaucoma 1, 3–4, 9, 70, 87
 – cause 71–2
 – coexistence with macular
  degeneration 5
 – driving 85–6
 – types 71–3, 74
 – what it is 70–1
 – see also angle-closure
  glaucoma; open-angle
  glaucoma
Great Ormond Street
  Hospital for Children
  NHS Trust 126–7
guide dogs 118
Guide Dogs for the Blind
  Association 127

hairwashing after cataract
  surgery 64
haptics 47
hard drusen 101
heart disease 79
help, where to find it
 – benefits and allowances
  118
 – in macular degeneration
  110
 – searching the internet
  133–5
 – useful addresses 123–32

high blood pressure 26
hospital admission, in angle-closure glaucoma 85
hospital eye service 8, 28–9
Housing Benefit 120
hydroxychloroquine, link to macular damage 102
hypermetropia (long-sightedness) 23
– association with glaucoma 83
– treatment 29, 30
hyphaema 93

Income Support 120
income tax, personal allowance 120
infections
– after surgery 65, 94
– treatment before surgery 55, 94
inflammation of the eye 65
inner chamber 17–19
inpatient cataract surgery 58
Institute of Child Health 127
intracapsular cataract surgery 49–51
intraocular lens implantation 2–3, 44, 46, 47
– after intracapsular cataract surgery 49, 51
– selection of lens 53–4
intraocular pressure (IOP) 71, 76
– measurement (tonometry) 77
– ocular hypertension 72–3
– see also glaucoma
iris 13, 14, 15, 18
– effect of prostaglandin drops 80

iritis 36
– after cataract surgery 65

lacrimal canal 11
lacrimal glands 11
laser surgery
– laser trabeculoplasty (LTP) 89
– for macular degeneration 108–9
– for open-angle glaucoma 89, 91, 92
– peripheral iridotomy 85, 86
– photodynamic therapy 112–14
– for posterior capsule opacification 66, 67
– for refractive errors 31–2
latanoprost 79
lens 13, 14, 16–17, 18, 39
– see also cataracts
lens implants 47
– selection 53–4
– see also intraocular lens implantation
lens replacement 2–3
– see also intraocular lens implantation
lenses for glasses 27–8
lethargy, as side effect of medication 80
levobunolol 80
lifting, avoidance after surgery 63, 95
lighting 122
local anaesthetics 59
long-sightedness (hypermetropia) 23
– association with glaucoma 83
– treatment 29, 30

LOOK, National Federation of Families with Visually Impaired Children 127
low vision aids 119
Lucentis (ranibizumab) 107–8
lutein 107

macula 18, 98, 99
macular degeneration 1, 4–5, 9, 116
  – age-related 100–1
    – causes 101
    – diagnosis 104–5
    – symptoms 103–4
    – treatment 105, 107–9, 112–15
    – who is affected 103
  – driving 112
  – getting help 110
  – glasses 119
  – long-term outlook 115
  – monitoring 109–10, 111
  – risk factors 102–3
  – what it is 98–9
Macular Disease Society 128
macular dystrophies 102
macular oedema (water logging) 65
medications
  – link to macular damage 102–3
  – review before cataract surgery 56–7, 60
  – as trigger for acute glaucoma 83
metipranolol 80
miotic eyedrops 80–1
mistiness of vision 38, 40
multifocal lens implants 54
muscles of eye 12, 13
myopia (short-sightedness) 23

  – association with other eye conditions 5, 75, 103
  – treatment 29, 30, 31

nasolacrimal duct 11
National Institute for Health and Clinical Excellence (NICE) 128
nausea, in angle-closure glaucoma 84
needling 94, 96
newspapers, talking 119, 132
NHS Direct 128, 134
NHS Smoking Helplines 128–9
nuclear sclerotic cataracts 37
  – symptoms 40
nurse practitioners 7

objective refraction test 27
occipital cortex 20
ocular hypertension 72–3
open-angle glaucoma 71, 72, 74, 87
  – causes 73
  – diagnosis 76–8
  – long-term monitoring 82–3
  – medical treatment 78–82
  – risk factors 75
  – surgery 88, 97
    – anaesthetics 94–5
    – benefits and risks 91, 92–4
    – laser treatment 89, 91, 92
    – postoperative recovery and treatment 95–6
    – questions to ask your consultant 93
    – trabeculectomy 88–9, 90
  – symptoms 75–6
  – see also glaucoma

ophthalmologists (ophthalmic surgeons) 5–6
ophthalmoscopy 76, 77
optic nerve 14, 18, 20
– cupping 76
optometrists 6, 26, 28
orthoptists 7
outpatient appointments, postoperative 62

pain, in angle-closure glaucoma 84
pain relief after surgery 62
partial sight, registration 117–18
Patients' Association 129
perimetry 78
peripheral blood vessel disease 80
peripheral iridotomy 85, 86, 89
personal income tax allowance 120
phacoemulsification 45–7, 69
photodynamic therapy (PDT) 112–14
photoreceptors 18, 19, 20
pilocarpine 80, 84
postage concessions 120
posterior capsule opacification 65–6, 67
posterior subcapsular cataracts 38
premedication, cataract surgery 59
preoperative assessment
– cataract surgery 55–6
– surgery for open-angle glaucoma 94
presbyopia 23, 32
pressure, raised see glaucoma

prostaglandin eyedrops 79–80
pupils 14
– adaptation to light levels 13, 15
– dilation for cataract surgery 60
– dilation for eye examination 52, 105

Quit (Smoking Quitlines) 129

radiation, as cause of cataracts 36
radiotherapy, for macular degeneration 114
railcards 121
rainbow effect around lights 83
ranibizumab (Lucentis) 107–8
reading glasses 32
reading lamps 122
red eye, angle-closure glaucoma 84
refraction tests 27
refractive errors 23
– correction by artificial lenses 53–4
– treatment 29–32
registration as blind or partially sighted 117–18
– benefits 120–1
retina 14, 18, 19
retinal pigment epithelial (RPE) cells, loss of 100
retinal translocation 115
retinoscope refraction test 27
rheumatoid arthritis medication, link to macular damage 102
Ridley, Harold 3, 44
rod photoreceptors 18, 19

Royal College of Ophthalmologists **130**

Royal National Institute of Blind People (RNIB) **118, 130–1**

rubella (German measles) **35**

scanning laser ophthalmoscope **77**

sclera **12, 14**

secondary glaucoma **73**

Sense **131–2**

shadows in field of vision **41**

short-sightedness (myopia) **23**
- association with other eye conditions **5, 75, 103**
- treatment **29, 30, 31**

side effects
- of alpha-2 agonists **82**
- of beta-blocker eyedrops **80**
- of carbonic anhydrase inhibitors **81**
- of miotic eyedrops **80–1**
- of prostaglandin eyedrops **79–80**
- of sympathomimetic eyedrops **81**
- of trabeculectomy **93**

sleepiness, as side effect of medication **80**

slit-lamp examination **41, 53**

small incision non-phacoemulsification cataract surgery (SICS) **47**

smoking
- as cause of cataracts **36**
- NHS Smoking Helplines **128–9**
- Quit (Smoking Quitlines) **129**

- risk of age-related macular degeneration **102, 107**

Snellen charts **24–6**

Social Services **117**

soft drusen **101**

specialist nurses **7**

steroids
- for angle-closure glaucoma **85**
- as cause of cataracts **36, 38**

stitches, removal after cataract surgery **63**

straining, avoidance after surgery **63, 95**

subjective refraction test **27**

subretinal neovascular membrane *see* wet-form age-related macular degeneration

sunlight exposure, as cause of cataracts **36**

surgery
- for open-angle glaucoma **97**
  - anaesthetics **94–5**
  - benefits and risks **91, 92–4**
  - laser treatment **89, 91, 92**
  - postoperative recovery and treatment **95–6**
  - preoperative assessment **94**
  - questions to ask your consultant **93**
  - trabeculectomy **88–9, 90, 91**
- peripheral iridotomy **85, 86**
- *see also* cataract surgery; laser surgery

suspensory ligaments
(zonules) **14, 16–17, 39**
sympathomimetic eyedrops
81

talking books and
newspapers **119**
– Calibre Cassette Library
124–5
– RNIB Talking Books
Service **130**
Talking Newspaper
Association UK (TNAUK)
132
tamoxifen, link to macular
damage **102**
tamsulosin hydrochloride
56–7
tax credits **118**
tear ducts **12**
tears **11–12**
telephone costs, assistance
121
Telephones for the Blind fund
121
timolol **80**
tingling, as side effect of
medication **81, 82**
tonometry **77**
topical anaesthesia **59**
trabecular meshwork **16, 71,
74**
trabeculectomy **88–9, 90**
– combination with
cataract surgery **91**
– pros and cons **93–4**
transport concessions **121**
trauma
– as cause of cataracts **36**
– as cause of macular
degeneration **102**
travoprost **79**

trifocal lenses **28**
TV licence **120**

uveitis **36**
– after cataract surgery **65**
uveoscleral pathway **71**

varifocal lenses **27**
vascular disease **79, 80**
vision
– effect of open-angle
glaucoma **75–6**
– recovery after cataract
surgery **61**
visual acuity tests **24–6**
visual cortices **20–1**
visual field loss, glaucoma **76**
visual fields **20–1**
– assessment (perimetry) **78**
vitamin supplements, in
macular degeneration
107
vitreous humour **14, 17, 19**
– removal during cataract
surgery **64**
vomiting, in angle-closure
glaucoma **84**

waiting lists, cataract surgery
42
Wales Council for the Blind
132
warfarin dose, cataract
surgery **56**
water logging (macular
oedema), after cataract
surgery **65**
wet-form age-related
macular degeneration
100–1, 110
– argon-laser therapy
108–9

- photodynamic therapy 112–14
- radiotherapy 114
- ranibizumab (Lucentis) treatment 107–8
- retinal translocation 115
- *see also* macular degeneration

'white of the eye' 12

zeaxanthin 107
zinc supplements, in macular degeneration 107
zonules (suspensory ligaments) 14, 16–17, 39

Your pages

We have included the following pages because they may help you manage your illness or condition and its treatment.

Before an appointment with a health professional, it can be useful to write down a short list of questions of things that you do not understand, so that you can make sure that you do not forget anything.

Some of the sections may not be relevant to your circumstances.

We are always pleased to receive constructive criticism or suggestions about how to improve the books. You can contact us at:

Email: familydoctor@btinternet.com
Letter   Family Doctor Publications
         PO Box 4664
         Poole
         BH15 1NN

Thank you

Health-care contact details

Name:

Job title:

Place of work:

Tel:

Name:

Job title:

Place of work:

Tel:

Name:

Job title:

Place of work:

Tel:

Name:

Job title:

Place of work:

Tel:

Significant past health events – illnesses/ operations/investigations/treatments

Event	Month	Year	Age (at time)

Appointments for health care

Name:

Place:

Date:

Time:

Tel:

Name:

Place:

Date:

Time:

Tel:

Name:

Place:

Date:

Time:

Tel:

Name:

Place:

Date:

Time:

Tel:

Appointments for health care

Name:

Place:

Date:

Time:

Tel:

Name:

Place:

Date:

Time:

Tel:

Name:

Place:

Date:

Time:

Tel:

Name:

Place:

Date:

Time:

Tel:

Current medication(s) prescribed by your doctor

Medicine name:

Purpose:

Frequency & dose:

Start date:

End date:

Medicine name:

Purpose:

Frequency & dose:

Start date:

End date:

Medicine name:

Purpose:

Frequency & dose:

Start date:

End date:

Medicine name:

Purpose:

Frequency & dose:

Start date:

End date:

Other medicines/supplements you are taking, not prescribed by your doctor

Medicine/treatment:

Purpose:

Frequency & dose:

Start date:

End date:

Medicine/treatment:

Purpose:

Frequency & dose:

Start date:

End date:

Medicine/treatment:

Purpose:

Frequency & dose:

Start date:

End date:

Medicine/treatment:

Purpose:

Frequency & dose:

Start date:

End date:

Questions to ask at appointments
(Note: do bear in mind that doctors work under great time pressure, so long lists may not be helpful for either of you)

Questions to ask at appointments
(Note: do bear in mind that doctors work under great time
pressure, so long lists may not be helpful for either of you)

Notes

Notes

Notes

Notes

Notes